PATHWAYS
TO PLEASURE

PATHWAYS TO PLEASURE

The Consciousness & Chemistry of Optimal Living

Harvey Milkman
Stanley Sunderwirth

LEXINGTON BOOKS
An Imprint of Macmillan, Inc.
NEW YORK

Maxwell Macmillan Canada
TORONTO

Maxwell Macmillan International
NEW YORK OXFORD SINGAPORE SYDNEY

Library of Congress Cataloging-in-Publication Data

Milkman, Harvey
    Pathways to pleasure : the consciousness & chemistry of optimal
living / Harvey Milkman and Stanley Sunderwirth.
        p.   cm.
ISBN 0–02–921273–1
1. Self-actualization (Psychology)   2. Conduct of life.
3. Pleasure. 4. Health.   I. Sunderwirth, Stanley G.   II. Title.
BF637.S4M544   1993
158′.1—dc20   93–22399
                                                                          CIP

Lexington Books
An Imprint of Macmillan, Inc.
866 Third Avenue, New York, N. Y. 10022

Maxwell Macmillan Canada, Inc.
1200 Eglinton Avenue East
Suite 200
Don Mills, Ontario M3C 3N1

Macmillan, Inc. is part of the Maxwell Communication
Group of Companies.

Printed in the United States of America

printing number
1   2   3   4   5   6   7   8   9   10

To our children

Tasha and Arielle
—Harvey B. Milkman

Arliss, Caleb, Stanley, and Eric
—Stanley G. Sunderwirth

You must do the things you think you cannot do.
—*Eleanor Roosevelt*

Contents

STAGE II

Skill Development

STAGE III

Implementation

Tables and Figures

Tables

Figures

Preface

We are prepped to avoid temptation ad infinitum—no drugs, no sex, no cholesterol. Very little has been offered by way of *yes*. We have therefore written a guidebook on self-actualization—a descriptive volume for becoming engaged in pleasurable and creative pursuits while maintaining a steady fix on personal harmony and sense of purpose throughout the lifespan. The concept of *natural highs* is introduced as a means for achieving extended pleasure through activities that promote health and well-being.

Guided by the Personal Pleasure Inventory (PPI) and other personality-probing tools, readers learn to practice a style of pleasure-seeking that fits their individual needs and can be used to develop greater intimacy, fulfilling projects, and a healthier lifestyle. *Pathways to Pleasure* invites readers to discover their own lifelong path to joy and fulfillment.

Drawing on current research in human development and the growing field of neurobiology, the underlying premise of *Pathways To Pleasure* is that mere knowledge of what's good for you doesn't ensure optimal living. While the book examines and explains in clear, everyday language the roles of psychology and brain chemistry in all pleasurable activities, we also devote considerable attention to the skills and attitudes necessary to deepen and intensify the abilities to relax, create, and enjoy. Intimate and caring relationships allow us to greet life's inevitable changes with celebration and grace.

PATHWAYS
TO PLEASURE

Introduction

Say Yes to Natural Highs

If I had my influence with the good fairy who is supposed to preside over the christening of all children I should ask that her gift to each child in the world would be a sense of wonder so indestructible that it would last throughout life, as an unfailing antidote against the boredom and disenchantment of later years, the sterile preoccupation with things that are artificial, the alienation from the sources of our strength.

—Rachel Carson, The Sense of Wonder

At some point in our adult lives, all of us have longed to be children again. We may regard this feeling as a twinge of nostalgia, easily dismissed, or as a genuine sadness at the passing of innocence. In any case, we are accustomed to looking at childhood as a simpler, happier time, certainly simpler than anything that follows in our journey in this world. It isn't just that children don't have to contend with all the challenges and pressures of adult life—the rat race at the office, the emotional and financial responsibilities of marriage and parenting, the complex tug-of-war involved in our various quests for love, friendship, success, status, spiritual fulfillment, and whatever else we think we're after. No, it isn't what is absent from childhood, but what children seem to possess that we don't. The average, healthy child knows how to have fun.

Youth is filled with opportunities to sample a seemingly endless array of wonderful sensations. Even as infants, we learn instinctively to distinguish between pleasure and pain, to seek one and shun the other. As we grow older, we become increasingly adventurous in our search for pleasure. Children delight in tree-climbing, roller-coaster riding, and finger painting; they jump off swings, play hide-and-seek, giggle at puppets and clowns, and enter into wildly imaginative adventures of their own devising. Diverse as these activities quickly become, they all share a common bond. They all offer healthy pleasures, and that sensation of pleasure derives, in varying degrees of intensity, from natural changes in brain chemistry.

The role of brain chemistry in achieving even the simplest physical pleasures should not be underestimated. Self-induced dizziness, a universal behavior in toddlers, clearly suggests that one way to feel good is to feel different—by altering the chemistry of the brain. In *Intoxication: Life in Pursuit of Artificial Paradise,* Ronald Siegal points out that such attempts at "mind alteration" aren't confined to the human race; a number of animals, including nonhuman primates, deliberately seek out various psychoactive substances found in nature—presumably so they can feel "different," too. For example, elephants have been known to gorge themselves on fermented fruit to the point of intoxication, and certain species of birds often plummet out of trees after getting "stoned" on their favorite berries!

Of course, the human quest for pleasure doesn't take quite such a ridiculous form—or does it? As young people mature, the more innocent varieties of childish play begin to lose their savor. During the transition from childhood to adolescence, spontaneous expression becomes inhibited as we begin to compare ourselves with others. We take on a facade, shaped by the expectations of community, family, and friends. The self-renewing pleasures associated with exercise, relaxation, art, nature, imaginative play—and even our everyday interactions with other people—gradually shift to the kind of vicarious satisfaction many of us take in following the accomplishments of media heroes such as athletes, movie stars, and television talk-show hosts. Our sources of personal pleasure become more "sophisticated" and, in many cases, more furtive: they include not only the joys of sex but the passive absorption of eating, shopping, and watching TV—and the potent effects of alcohol and drugs. One recent national survey indicates that by the time they have become high school seniors, 90 percent of our children have used alcohol, nearly 50 percent have smoked marijuana, and 40 percent have tried cocaine.

For many adolescents, this encounter with mind-altering chemicals will turn out to be merely a flirtation, an experiment. But for others, it will become a lifelong struggle with substance abuse, a struggle that is all too familiar to thousands of drug addicts and millions of alcoholics. The process of addiction defies simple explanation, just as it defies social expectation. When children are asked if they would choose to become alcoholics or drug addicts, they nearly always view the question as absurd: "Of course not!" Yet nearly 25 percent of our population suffers from one or more compulsive problem behaviors. How does the huge discrepancy between childhood idealism and adult desperation arise?

Certainly there has been no shortage of warnings about false paradise. Throughout the history of Western civilization, from the time of Hammurabi's Code to our own narcotics statutes, the laws and standards of human conduct have been riddled with injunctions against the use or abuse of certain substances. Even in ancient cultures, overindulgence in alcohol, sex, or food was frequently condemned. Our own society has a vast (if somewhat less than effective) tradition of seeking to battle addiction by controlling or banishing the substance in question. Just as the Puritans railed against tobacco and Carrie Nation sought to stem the flow of demon rum, so has the federal government sought to enlist the entire country in its "war" on crack cocaine.

The war on drugs, like most campaigns against addiction, seems to rise and fall depending on prevailing social attitudes. We move through cycles of tolerance and intolerance, establishing a national prohibition of alcohol and then repealing it, decriminalizing marijuana in one decade and recriminalizing it in the next. Ironically, at the moment the pendulum has swung far to the side of intolerance (or "zero tolerance") with respect to the drug problem. Nancy Reagan's campaign to get kids to "Just Say No" to drugs has become the battle cry for any number of causes: no drunk driving, no casual sex, no teenage pregnancy, no rap music. Indeed, it is no exaggeration to suggest that the prevailing message our leaders are beaming to us is a big flashing NO, reminiscent of the kinds of signs one sees in subways and public buildings: NO—Eating/Smoking/Spitting/Alcoholic Beverages/Loitering/Ball Playing/or Dogs.

No doubt about it, we are prepped to avoid temptation ad infinitum. Why, then, do so many young people still become casualties in the war on drugs? Why do so many of them develop terrible dependencies on drugs, alcohol, or destructive forms of behavior (e.g., compulsive overeating) that dog them through adulthood and may actually shorten their lives?

Obviously, part of the answer is that knowledge alone—urging kids to "Just Say No" and providing detailed information on the dangers of smoking crack or drinking oneself into a stupor—isn't sufficient to deter people from destructive pleasure-seeking. If knowledge were the key ingredient, then people who drive cars would always wear seatbelts, newfound lovers would insist that their partners get tested for sexually transmitted diseases (STDs) before going to bed with them, and intravenous drug users would never share needles. Health information is effective only when received by a person fully equipped with what might be described as the emotional and behavioral "competencies" to act on that knowledge. Unfortunately, many people don't seem to develop such competencies, except through bitter experience, if at all.

This book offers a connoisseur's approach to enhancing pleasure in everyday life—without drugs, harmful addictive behaviors, or simplistic "recipes for feeling good" (e.g., get aerobic, meditate, eat your oat bran). Drawing on current research in developmental and self psychology, personal accounts of people who have made contact with their "creative spirit," and the growing field of brain chemistry (five-year-old Tasha recently told a group of adults that "the brain works the body, and it works itself, too"), this volume presents a guide to becoming meaningfully engaged in one's unique proclivities for learning, productivity, and self-expression while maintaining a steady fix on personal harmony and sense of purpose through the lifespan.

Alan Dumas, feature writer for the *Rocky Mountain News,* was given the assignment to write about people who are just ordinary, yet interesting in their personal means to maintain well-being through unique forms of self-expression. This book is written for readers who, like Dumas's interviewees, are seeking a greater sense of fulfillment throughout their lives, but are not necessarily committed to becoming recognized for their extraordinary talents or physical abilities. In fact, a central lesson from his inquiry into the lives of more than 250 "creative spirits" is to stop thinking about artistic expression in terms of gift or talent. Whether the product of our efforts is "good" or not is a subjective judgment, quite independent of the genuine fulfillment resulting from self-expression. According to Dumas, just about anybody who has the will to do so, and the confidence in themselves to do so, can enter into the creative process and be enriched by it. It is not something that is closed off to the talented or the beautiful or the powerful or the privileged. There are homeless people who are expressing themselves in a way that is very satisfying to them. There are all kinds of different people—old and young, rich and poor—nothing can stop the creative process when someone is determined to enter it.

Dumas found that people who are able to derive fulfillment from self-expression are not limited by traditional thinking about what constitutes a creative act—such as writing a book or playing a musical instrument. Some have discovered their creative centers privately, while others have found help in groups or organizations. A number have been thrust into the creative journey by personal crises, when dramatic changes such as a divorce, loss of a loved one, or retirement forced them to reconsider and restructure their patterns of existence, while others have simply started the creative process, without any apparent drama in their lives. Whatever the origin, the underlying thoughts and feelings are quite universal:

- I need to change my life.
- I want to uncover hidden feelings.
- There's something I want to contribute that is going unexpressed.

Consider Cindy Parker, who describes herself as a woman typical of her generation. At thirty-six, she has been married and divorced, is raising a teenage daughter, works as a secretary, and is not particularly well read. But she has always loved to write poetry and has dreamed of running her own business. She emerged from the mist of pure fantasy by combining her own romantic trials, her affinity for poetry, and her entrepreneurial drive. For the past four years, Parker has spent most of her spare time writing love poems for those too shy or uninspired to do so for themselves. Her special twist is that she doesn't strive to write good poetry; rather, she wants to write poetry that sounds like you or I (or whoever the client) composed it. She purposefully wrote this very ineloquent verse for a man who wanted something written for his wife's anniversary:

> For many years I have known you,
> you,
> You were the family who lived
> down the street
> But then one day I fell in love
> with
> The girl with the funny-looking
> feet.

Parker's biggest problem thus far has been marketing. After striking out with newspaper display ads, she's dropped more than 50,000 fliers and written about thirty-five poems that take her about twenty minutes each, for which she charges $35.00. Her latest scheme is to target truckers, who she realizes are on the road a lot and feel guilty about it, so she took an ad in *Truckers's News,* offering to send personalized notes to truckers' loved ones on a monthly basis for one year.

Walter Kranz, an insurance broker, World War II veteran, and successful advertising executive, retired from traditional work during his mid seventies. He then discovered what a lot of people have found—that in your seventies, if you don't go to work, you start to fade away pretty fast. Hard-driven businesspeople deteriorate rapidly and soon die. Walter Kranz knew enough about himself to know he was such a type. He decided to write a play.

Now, even the most naive would-be artists recognize that writing a play is one of the least likely forms of creativity to be recognized or appreciated. And even more strange and therefore delightful is that Walter Kranz decided to write about Warren G. Harding, whom he's old enough to remember as president from when he was a boy. As people now write about Jack Kennedy in the Camelot years, Kranz wrote about Harding during the twenties. Kranz took this obvious recipe for failure and made it work. He finished the play, found a director, and recruited an actor to play Warren G. Harding. He put it together, got a very credible production going, and started pushing it, at first to a local rotary club and civic groups, and then it traveled out of state. From just sheer energy and the determination to contribute, Kranz made this effort a successful venture. And if you asked him, he'd say, "The alternative was dying."

But most people—unlike Cindy Parker and Walter Kranz—don't

take on the creative challenge. Rather, they become seduced by some promise of false paradise. They succumb to a pattern of behavior that, because of its immediacy and flush of primary delight, becomes imprinted as a strategy for having fun. Whether drink, money, sex, cars, calories, or crack, people first recreationally, soon matter-of-factly, and later compulsively begin to binge on superficial props for feeling good.

Even if we accept that drug education can provide a deterrent in some instances, there is a larger, more basic mystery to the phenomenon of harmful pleasure-seeking. Most of us begin life with exquisite instincts for pleasure and play, a seemingly boundless capacity for love and happiness—and yet in those very qualities may lie the secret of our undoing. As we pass through the incredible journey from childhood to maturity, we experience an incessant hunger to retain the spontaneity, luminosity, and joy of youth. As will be shown throughout this book, caring relationships and steady guidance through the transitions of life can make all the difference between health and depredation. Eloquently stated by W. Somerset Maugham, "The road to salvation is narrow and difficult to walk, like the razor's edge."

The phrase "rites of passage" is used to describe the colorful array of rituals and ceremonies that serve to ease the transition from one status or role to another, across the lifespan—to soften the "razor's edge." If, for whatever reason, these orienting systems fail, humans will gravitate toward whatever they can grasp as they struggle to maintain balance amid the storm and stress of significant life changes. Whether gang initiation, ritualized drug use, immersion in higher education, adventurous world travel, or completion of a religious pilgrimage, rites of passage have three common elements: (1) *separation*—a clear departure from the former status; (2) *transition*—a period of learning new customs or expectations; and (3) *reintroduction*—a return to life in the new status, marked by a series of rituals.

Consider the following excerpts from one teenager's story of a passage from innocence to experience. Mary Barnes, a twenty-one-year-old college student and aspiring actress, has reclaimed her personality after a tormenting interlude of drug abuse. This account of one young woman's descent into drugs and return to creativity is offered as a metaphor for a rite of passage into the realm of self-actualization. In some—those relatively few who emerge un-scathed—a drug interlude represents a *threshold period,* character-ized by disorientation and emotional unrest. The journey to self-dis-covery reaches a turning point when one severs from former obstacles to creativity, such as unhealthy family ties or other social encumbrances. The traveler returns at a more integrated level, fi-nally tapping into his or her channels for self-expression, so natural to children who are free to be themselves.

> All of the neighborhood kids would gather on the street for a game of hide-and-seek. We had water-balloon fights, carnivals, lemonade stands, all sorts of clubs, and a lot of fun. Yet I was always indepen-dent and would spend time alone feeding the ducks or building sand castles or reading a book. The days were seemingly endless. . . . When high school came, my life began its downward spiral. My brother had been doing drugs for a while. . . . More pressure was put on me to be everything he was not. . . . I started going to parties, discovered alco-hol, and became such a cute, innocent drunk. I wanted to be popular; I wanted everyone to like me; I needed attention. After I stayed out all night once too often, my parents gave me the ultimatum: shape up or ship out. I got an apartment the next day. Now I could do whatever I pleased.

In Mary's case, "whatever I pleased" turned out to be not very pleasant at all. Her youthful drug experimentation degenerated into an expensive cocaine habit that caused her to drop out of school and soon threatened her very existence.

> After four months of using cocaine on a regular basis, I found myself horribly ill, unable to keep anything down, throwing up blood, and doubled over with stomach pain. I called my mom and she took me to the hospital, where I spent a week being probed and prodded. A bleeding ulcer was diagnosed, and I was sent on my way with a spe-cial diet. Since I had decided it was a dog-eat-dog world, I took some money and ran. It was only five grand. . . . I heard that the people looking for me planned to take me up to the mountains, tie me up, pour gasoline over me, and set me on fire. Desperate, my parents bribed me with cash and a horse to check into a drug treatment pro-gram in the wilderness of Montana. Those six weeks may have saved my life. First, I endured a survival course out in the middle of no-where. We hiked twenty to thirty miles a day. I boiled water in order

to drink it and fasted for up to three days before earning a bag of flour, peanuts, and raisins. Being stripped of all my defenses helped me to realize that I didn't want to live the way I was living anymore. I cried long and hard for the first time in years as my soul began to cleanse itself. The next three weeks, we went rock-climbing, kayaking, and mountain-climbing. We had frequent group meetings, and I surrendered fully to them. All the parents came up at the end for a huge, emotional reunion. . . . I stayed on at boarding school for another nine months and dealt with many issues from the past, such as my adoption and need for perfection. I was able to accept myself completely for the first time in my life. I was learning to trust other people and developed the foundation for an open, honest relationship with my parents. . . . I learned there that not everyone was going to be my friend, like me, and approve of me. The fact that I had a drug problem and was verifiably an addict came to light. I learned a lot about addictions and was able to come to grips with my use and abuse and how it affected my life so severely. . . . I left with a deep appreciation for nature, a peaceful inner feeling, and a passionate lust for life.

Sounds wonderful, doesn't it? Mary left the treatment program convinced that she had conquered her demons and was ready to start living a "passionate," drug-free life. But she soon discovered that her bout with addiction was far from over.

All my old friends were anxiously waiting for me so they could party. It took me a long time to learn that if I hang around drugs, I'm sucked right in. I even started smoking cigarettes again, after I had gone through the torture of quitting five months earlier. . . . I quit my job and went back to selling LSD; it was so much easier and provided a much higher income—up to $1,000 on a good day. . . . I would work on location at concerts and parties, living life in the fast lane eighteen hours a day. Whenever I used cocaine, I was completely out of control, having to smoke a ton of pot and drink more alcohol than an alcoholic would, just to take the edge off coming down. I was miserable. I would vow never to do it again. I would tell people not to give it to me, even if I begged. But then the next day would come, fresh and new, and I'd start all over again. I hadn't lost hope of making something of my life, though, and enrolled in school again. I had a wonderful psychology teacher, who may well have influenced my decision to pursue it. But more than likely, I enjoyed it so much because of all the psychological bullshit I've experienced firsthand. . . . I entered my first horse show in almost three years. Although my performance was only passable, I was doing something for me and no one else. At the next big show, we made champion. . . . I broke up with my boyfriend, whose interests remained getting high and playing the guitar, while mine were growing into horse training and school. I continued to win throughout that summer. Each time the awards were announced, I felt renewed, a sense of pride and joy beyond any imaginable feeling. . . . I went to work at the riding academy again and loved working with the kids. Meanwhile, my war with cocaine continued. I still had a daily habit and weighed under ninety pounds. . . . One morning, I woke up determined to make it to my class despite the lingering effects of Valium. I reached the bathroom and was horrified by the haggard, old, and sick reflection in the mirror of the person I called myself. As I stared at her eye to eye, tears ran down her face, over the bags, over the puffy cheeks, down. Shocked and scared, I crawled back to bed, resolving that I couldn't go on like this anymore. I had reached the end of my rope. . . . The following morning, I went in to talk with the instructor of my "Cravings and Addictions" class. I was able to use his support and commit to not using drugs, one day at a time. I slowly got free. During the next two months, I used very seldom. . . . I put more effort into school, excelling academically. I went to Hawaii with my family and had a great time. I was finally happy. I went to work at a flower and gardening shop for the remainder of the year. I thoroughly enjoyed my work and took pride in learning all about the plants and flowers. Everything was more fun: concerts, riding, my family, and even waking up in the morning. I played on a volleyball team, at about the same time that I quit smoking for good. . . . In my first year of sobriety, I changed dramatically. I looked different, younger, and, ironically enough, innocent. My morals were higher, as my self-esteem had doubled. I could think clearly; it was as if my brainpower had actually increased. I would soar through my classes easily. I behaved differently, too. I was so comfortable with myself that I could be open, honest, and loving with people. . . . There is no longer a bottomless hole inside me, desperately needing to be filled. I am enough. Natural highs have taken the place of artificial ones. Every day, I have peak experiences, riding, skiing, performing, listening to music, or enjoying a beautiful sunset. I live each day as if it were my last.

Although Mary's account is primarily the story of her personal voyage to self-discovery, it contains several elements common to countless others. We've all heard such stories (or confessions) at one time or another—but have we really understood them?

Let's begin with the process by which Mary became acquainted with drugs in the first place. Mary insists her childhood was a happy one, and we have no reason to doubt her. She played games and enjoyed being close to her family and friends. She also had a distinct sense of individuality. Contrary to popular belief, harmful pleasure-seeking does not always have its roots in early childhood and dysfunctional families. Still, when her older brother began using drugs, Mary's need to imitate, compete, and win peer approval led her down a similar path. She became a "cute, innocent drunk," and apparently a popular one, too. In the rush to urge kids to reject drugs, this is a point that is often overlooked—the power of "peer pressure" and related factors holds much greater sway over most adolescents than parental authority, and the messages one receives from one's peers may be quite at odds with (and far more persuasive than) "Just Say No."

As in the Japanese proverb "The man takes a drink, the drink takes a drink, the drink takes the man," Mary's identity revolved around drugs, to the exclusion of just about everything else. Left to her own devices, she succeeded at being a loser. Mary soon reached what is known in the self-help community as "incomprehensible demoralization." She committed crimes, dropped out of school, and spit blood. Her parents were forced to show their concern through the only means left—so-called tough love.

The turning point came when Mary entered treatment in the Montana wilderness. Through a series of new relationships, she learned skills, attitudes, and self-expectations that allowed her to cross into adulthood. She became interested in understanding the origins of her problems, while beginning to accept personal responsibility for her actions ("I was able to accept myself completely for the first time. . . . I learned there that not everyone was going to be my friend, like me, and approve of me").

The lure of previous haunts, though, is compelling. Despite the fact that she had begun to acquire a new understanding of herself, Mary's relapse was probably inevitable; she had yet to acquire new ways of coping with everyday existence back in the "real world" (as opposed to a rustic retreat in Montana) without using drugs. But by pursuing her innate talents and interests—horses, scholarship, athletics, gardening, performing—and with the support of the close personal relationships she had developed, she was able to build a strong foundation for recovery.

Both of these factors, the personal relationships and the growing involvement in productive activities, are essential to Mary's story. Without the care and steadfast support of her teachers and parents, it is doubtful she could have survived; but with their help, and after a year of savoring what she calls "natural highs" and "peak experiences," Mary is well insulated against the continued seduction of false paradise. This last point can't be too strongly stressed. One of the most common criticisms of the "Just Say No" approach is that it doesn't give children something to say yes to—at least, not something that is as appealing to curious, vulnerable young people as the lure of drugs. Therapists who work with recovering drug addicts talk about the need for "alternative gratification," but most drug prevention programs devote more attention to the horrors of drug abuse than to exploring alternatives that might help a person, as the cliché has it, to "get high on life." (One program in a Colorado school system urges kids to "Say Yes to Homework," but it seems unlikely that most students will find a couple of hours of algebra all that gratifying.) Yet as Mary's story illustrates, positive substitutes for drugs are necessary if we are to steer clear of the "bottomless hole" of substance abuse. Saying yes to new, healthy experiences is what *Pathways to Pleasure* is all about. Drawing on the lessons from Mary and others, this book offers a rational strategy for optimal living.

Our discussion begins with a fundamental source of human unrest: the relentless urge to feel wonderful. Consider a recent discussion between the legendary cartoon characters Calvin and Hobbes:

[Calvin (boy) leads Hobbes (toy tiger) on a breathtaking wagon ride through hill and dale.]

CALVIN: Life is like topography, Hobbes. There are summits of happiness and success; . . . Flat stretches of boring routine . . . and valleys of frustration and failure . . . but *I'm* dedicating myself to experiencing only *peaks!* I want my life to be one never ending ascension! . . . Each minute should bring me greater joy than the previous minute. . . . I should always be saying "my life is better than I ever imagined it would be, and it's only going to improve." . . . I'm just going to jump from peak to peak! I'm . . . *whoops*. . . .

[Calvin misdirects the speeding wagon carrying Hobbes and himself off the edge of a steep cliff. The last bit of conversation occurs while the two are tumbling in midair.]

HOBBES: At least with flat places you don't have so far to go down.

CALVIN: Only *losers* go down! For me it's only going to be *up* and *up!*

The cartoon is effective because it speaks to a collective unconscious. The desire to have *more* of everything, to "experience only peaks," is a basic impulse of the human psyche. For many people, the anxiety associated with this persistent and dangerous urge to outdo previous experience—to feel better than the time before—becomes diverted to a narrow focus on drugs and alcohol. Drinking and drugging then become the scapegoats for what is really a much deeper drive, best described as a *craving for ecstasy.*

The craving for ecstasy—the root cause of compulsive pleasure-seeking—springs from one's early encounters with pleasurable activities. Just as the toddler makes the discovery that spinning oneself into a dizzy heap can make the spinner feel good (by altering brain chemistry), the older child or adolescent sets out to get "hammered" on beer or high on marijuana, knowing this will produce an altered state of mind. It's the sensation of altered mood, the effect it produces—*not* the substance itself—that we crave. This fundamental verity of drug use is often overlooked as society's attention becomes increasingly focused on the drugs themselves as the evil source of our problems.

Our national war on drugs is based on the premise that illegal drug use can be reduced, or even eradicated, if we can successfully attack the means of supply (through border interdiction, prosecution of dealers, raids on crack houses, and other forms of law enforcement) and the level of demand (through drug education and treatment programs). Yet how can our efforts to reduce demand ever be successful unless we begin by trying to understand the chemistry of craving that leads people to take drugs in the first place?

We don't mean to imply that the current drug problem, in all its complexity, simply boils down to how drugs affect the brain. Clearly there are complex economic, sociological, and psychological factors involved in the spread of drug abuse across our land. Still, the current debate raging over if, when, or how society will deal with psychoactive substances—Is drug addiction a disease, or a bad habit? Can some people use drugs recreationally? Should society legalize certain mood-altering substances, or ban those which are still tolerated, such as alcohol and tobacco—begs a much larger question, not about drugs, but about the nature of pleasure.

Consider the implications of Mary's story again. If we accept that her descent into addiction began as an extension of her youthful pursuit of pleasure, of "peak experiences," then there is an interesting corollary in her recovery. The same hunger that spurred on her desperate embrace of cocaine—the craving for ecstasy, the drive to get high—can also lead to natural highs that are not only physically beneficial but deeply satisfying on an emotional and spiritual level in a way drugs never can be.

Providing a Positive Direction for Mood Alteration

In the seminars we have developed that explore the concept of natural highs, we have occasionally encountered well-meaning educators and health professionals who are deeply uncomfortable with the notion of promoting any kind of "highs," natural or otherwise. As they see it, getting high—with all its implications of mood alteration, self-gratification, and escape from the everyday world—is essentially an irresponsible act. How, they wonder, can we ever mount an effective drug prevention campaign if we're still urging young people to get high on *anything?* Such misgivings are understandable. To some extent, they are even shared by some of the self-help gurus who tell audiences to "get high on life"; whatever it is they are recommending (a joyful acceptance of everyday existence?), they surely aren't advocating fooling around with brain chemistry. "Getting high" is loaded language, a phrase that smacks of the drug culture of the 1960s and all its terrors. (Back in 1968, when the rock group The Doors appeared on "The Ed Sullivan Show," the term was regarded as so sinister that singer Jim Morrison was asked to substitute another lyric for the line "Girl, we couldn't get much higher" in the hit song "Light My Fire." Morrison sang the line as written, and The Doors were banned from future appearances on the television show.)

Our response to these objections is to encourage seminar participants to take a broader view of the process of mood alteration and its possible benefits. Not every self-induced change in brain chemistry is necessarily wrong or harmful. (In fact, some changes are not only desirable but inevitable, such as the flood of adrenalin that enables us to cope with a sudden trauma or shock, a circumstance that will be discussed in detail in Chapter 3: The Chemical Brain.)

Perhaps discomfort with the notion of natural highs stems from our contradictory social attitudes toward pleasure itself. On the one hand, much of our lives is devoted to the quest to feel wonderful, even if it means engaging in self-destructive behavior; yet few of us would admit that the pursuit of pleasure is one of our top priorities. That would make us "hedonists," a term that once referred to followers of an ancient ethic of pleasure, but these days conjures up images of a shabby libertine, a dope-smoking "swinger" of questionable morals and judgment. Our heritage, from biblical times to the days of the dour Puritans, is full of admonitions that we should subordinate our need for pleasure to a higher good, indicating that there is something petty, even regressive, in our desire for personal enjoyment. "When I became a man, I put aside childish things," St. Paul said (1 Cor. 13:11). Many of us, in our desire to be mature, serious members of adult society, see our early discovery of mood-altering experiences as one of those "childish things" to be put aside rather than cultivated.

The "natural highs" concept implies that we *should* cultivate such experiences, for our own health and sense of well-being. Provocative as the term might seem, natural highs are simply ways to feel good through healthy alterations of brain chemistry. In an article entitled "The Chemistry of Craving," first published in *Psychology Today* in 1983, we defined addiction as "self-induced changes in neurotransmission that result in problem behaviors." Natural highs originate in similar changes but with dramatically different results; thus, a definition readily follows:

Natural highs: Self-induced changes in brain chemistry that result in optimal living.

In other words, natural highs are feelings of pleasure that are triggered by healthy activities.

If we subscribe to a traditional, Western view of "health" as the absence of disease, then the idea of getting "high" to get healthy may seem somewhat bizarre. But increasingly, physicians and researchers are coming to the realization that there's more to a truly healthy life than a body free of tumors. The World Health Organization had defined health as "a state of complete physical, mental and social well-being and not merely the absence of disease or infirmity." The attainment of well-being involves toning the mental outlook as well as the muscles, and healing social wounds as well as personal ones. Natural highs can be a vital tool in implementing this broader, more positive agenda for a healthy society. Considering the specter of addiction facing so many of our young people, the need for such a tool is great. Health promotion and drug prevention responsibilities can no longer be shunted to school personnel or law enforcement officials. True, part of the solution requires a concerted effort to provide early education—at home and in the classroom—about the dangers associated with drugs. We must, however, be aware that such information might arouse a child's curiosity and sense of adventure. A young person might even choose to experiment with the very substance he or she discovers through a school presentation on the dangers of drug abuse. Further, children might unearth other means of thrill-seeking, such as alcohol, automobile racing, or prostitution, not covered by narrowly defined prevention programs. By taking a positive approach to mood alteration—avoid undue emphasis on negative behaviors and abuse of illicit substances—the inconclusive debates on the relative dangers of drugs versus alcohol and the tedious admonitions about overindulgence in this or that behavior can be sidestepped. Most important, natural highs provide a positive way to manage brain chemistry in order to produce exhilaration devoid of anguish and calm without stupor, a process with applications well beyond the scope of drug prevention efforts. Through personal accounts, readers can see how real people incorporate natural highs into their lives. Consider excerpts from the journals of three ordinary people who have discovered their individual keys to pleasure and self-actualization:

Robert—

Through the day, tension builds up; one needs a release. Often I find that doing drawings or other artistic style helps me unwind. As I begin, the tension flows through my body, chest, neck, arms, all of them releasing the tension, and up into my mind. Here the stress is transformed and is released as it travels back through my arm and onto the paper. It's a fluid transgression, from tension to a form of bliss in which one finds calmness. Everything is still, and it's just you, your mind, and your talent at work.

Lynne—

When listening to music, I gain a sense of peace, a sense of well-being, a feeling of love for humanity, a feeling of confidence that any difficulty can be met with dignity. I find that my personal quiet time, spent with the music of my choice, is a daily necessity for me to be able to meet my family and work obligations in this fast-paced, complex world in which we live.

Iris—

Receiving the Challenger Award ranked alongside getting married to my husband and finding out I was going to be a mother. My face felt flushed and my heart was pounding. I felt as if my head was going to explode. I had such a happy grin that my mouth felt like it could crack! When it was my turn to speak about my future plans, I began to explode with tears of joy.

It is our hope that this book will prove useful to a wide spectrum of readers—parents, teachers, school administrators, law enforcement officials, students, and public policy makers—who are seeking to promote healthy alternatives to alcohol, drugs, or other harmful pleasure-inducing experiences. Still, *Pathways to Pleasure* isn't designed to be merely "educational" in the manner of a filmstrip or a class lecture. What follows is an invitation to develop the skills to experience your own natural highs, a sane and ultimately healthy way to tap into the well of ecstasy within that awaits each and every one of us.

1

Blueprint for Fulfillment

The most promising faith for the future might be based on the realiza-
tion that the entire universe is a system related by common laws and that
it makes no sense to impose our dreams and desires on nature without
taking them into account. Recognizing the limitations of human will,
accepting a cooperative rather than a ruling role in the universe, we
should feel the relief of the exile who is finally returning home. The
problem of meaning will then be resolved as the individual's purpose
merges with the universal flow.

—*Mihaly Csikzentmihalyi,* Flow: The Psychology
of Optimal Experience

The man holds an egg up to the camera.

"This," he says, "is your brain."

He cracks the shell and empties its contents into a hot skillet. The
egg begins to sizzle and pop.

"This is your brain on drugs," he says. "Get the picture?"

If you've watched any television in the past few years, you've
probably seen this public service announcement presented by the
Partnership for a Drug-Free America, not once, but several times.
The spot has generated considerable comment, including quite a few
snickers and groans from teenagers for its heavy-handedness. It has
even been parodied in a popular poster that depicts first a single
fried egg, then a hearty breakfast: "This is your brain on drugs. . . .
This is your brain on drugs with a side of bacon."

Parody aside, it's hard *not* to "get the picture" of drug use that the
man in the commercial wants us to get. Whether the spot has actually deterred any viewer from taking drugs is another matter. As we

noted earlier, knowledge alone isn't sufficient to keep kids off drugs; in fact, information about drugs, even when the information is presented in a negative context, can backfire. Multiple studies evaluating the efficiency of drug education classes among junior high school students found that those who took courses on the dangers of substance abuse used even more drugs than before they began the prevention program. The rise in drug use was possibly fueled by curiosity and the lure of risk-taking.

In other words, even if a child understands that drugs can "fry" the brain—and who can watch the egg demonstration and not understand that?—he or she might still cave in to curiosity and peer pressure. Knowledge is most effective when combined with the skills to act on that knowledge (e.g., having the social skills to cope with stressful situations without taking drugs).

The same holds true for natural highs. A thorough appreciation of the subject begins by understanding the causes and consequences of mood alteration, but *practiced skills* are a vital complement to sheer information. You can grasp the concept on an intellectual level, yet never experience what it offers unless you have prepared yourself for appropriate action. Our approach to *self-discovery* involves a kind of personal training program, with an organizational theme not unlike that found in Lamaze childbirth training. For a woman in labor, knowledge about what happens in utero pales in comparison to the application of coping skills she needs to make it through the next contraction. Lamaze students will forever value the pain-saving skills of relaxation, focal point, cleansing breath, and rhythmic breathing—ah hee . . . ah hee . . . ah hee . . . ah hoo!

To some extent, self-discovery is about relaxation and focal points, too. But it is also about choosing your own "type" of mood-altering activities, about raising healthy families, eating healthy food, cultivating intimacy and connectedness, and pursuing other endeavors designed to expand your capacity for healthy pleasures. The process is divided into three basic stages: mental preparation, skill development, and implementation. Each of these three stages will be addressed in detail in subsequent chapters. The following overview—a bird's-eye view of the terrain we'll be covering—should give you some idea of what to expect and help you get started.

Mental Preparation

We can depend on neither drugs nor good fortune for the experience of prolonged pleasure. As Abraham Lincoln quipped, "A person is as happy as his mind allows him to be." Mental preparation begins with cultivating a sense of optimism and a realistic attitude about feeling good.

Attitude has more to do with our general state of well-being than most of us realize. People who look on the bright side not only enjoy enthusiastic support from their friends and are able to better capitalize on opportunities for enjoyment as they arise, but also have more resistance to physical illness and depression. Suzanne Kobasa's work on the relationship between stress and illness is often cited in support of the notion that positive thinking can have an impact on the outcome of a given situation. She found that people under highly stressful life situations are able to overcome them, and in some cases actually thrive on them, because of their constructive attitude. Hardy individuals operate on the basis of three C's: commitment, challenge, and control.

When faced with dramatic changes, resilient people feel an increased determination to continue on behalf of themselves and their families. They view crisis as a challenge, rather than as a time for buckling under. Further, stress-resistant people maintain a belief— even to the point of illusion—that they can exert some degree of control over their situation.

In order to begin the journey of self-discovery, you might want to start by taking stock of your own attitudes about pleasure and suffering. In the face of adversity, are you more likely to "rise to the challenge" or to passively "ride out the storm," feeling you have no say in the matter? When was the last occasion you really took time out to enjoy yourself—and was the enjoyment tainted by a gnawing anxiety about the fact that good times don't last? If last night's social engagement had its share of pleasant and traumatic moments (as most do), are you haunted by the latter, or do you take comfort by reviewing the more enjoyable aspects of the experience? Whether you "light a candle" or "curse the darkness" can reveal a great deal about your capacity for pleasure.

When scientists measure the degree to which an individual feels happy or content, some interesting findings result. Despite the intellectual development attributable to evolution, we seem to share a common perception with prehistoric humans: we tend to gauge our happiness and security in relationship to the immediate past. If, for example, our ancestors were on the lookout for a saber-toothed tiger, happiness would be judged on the basis of perceived danger, not five years ago, but five minutes ago. This biological predisposition remains the determinant of modern humans' mood. Our sense of well-being is drawn from the effect of recent experiences, rather than major milestones in our lives. When nothing new happens, we tend to perceive life as unsatisfying, lackluster, and boring.

One way of cultivating an optimistic frame of mind is to compare your present situation not to yesterday's, but rather to how you were faring perhaps some time ago, when things weren't going so well. Of course, dwelling on past traumas or tragedies can be disquieting in itself; a brief reminder is all you'd want. But counting your blessings daily—being thankful for what is really going well in your life—is an important tool for feeling good.

When you consider the frenetic roar and sizzle that can be achieved by igniting one's mood with drugs, it is difficult to imagine that any natural activity could offer the same payoff. True, natural highs cannot compete with drugs in intensity. Rather, they can provide a foundation of gentle pleasures culminating in fulfillment and a sense of purpose throughout the lifespan. As Robert Ornstein and David Sobel eloquently point out in their book *Healthy Pleasures,* prolonged satisfaction does not hinge on the "big win":

> A life filled with many small moments of happiness—even simple ones such as playing hide and go seek with one's child, strapping on a portable cassette player and blotting out the delay of your plane's departure with your favorite Mozart, playing harmonica (even badly), trying to paint a landscape, or doing meaningful work—seems to deliver happiness. These small pleasures, whether they are sensual or mental, reading or roller-skating, can absorb some of the shocks and difficulties of life and contribute to ongoing happiness.

People who consider themselves genuinely happy are those who develop what Ornstein and Sobel have termed "a longing for repetition." They repetitiously seek, attain, and enjoy simple pleasures. These are not the sorts of jolts to the system one expects from drugs (or, if certain advertising campaigns are to be believed, from the consumption of a particular brand of soft drink). They are part of a subtler but ultimately more durable network of sensory delights, the enjoyment of which is enhanced rather than dulled by the memory of previous encounters of a similar nature. The joys of repetition are evident in the remarks of Meredith Fogg, an Australian living in the United States, in anticipation of a visit from her mother:

> Mum is lucky, 'cause when she comes to stay, the stone fruits will be out: cherries, apricots, peaches, and nectarines. She would have eaten them last Christmas and now summer again here, and in six months again at home. Three times in one year.

To a great extent, establishing the mental groundwork for self-discovery is a matter of reexamining and possibly redefining your attitudes and expectations. Moving from habitual pessimism to a self-confident enthusiasm for current challenges, from a restless quest for novelty or escape to a celebration of repeated pleasures, from a horror of boredom to a sense of wonder at the mysteries of everyday living—each step of "attitude adjustment" takes us closer to savoring those cherries and peaches the way they should be savored. And armed with our revived sense of wonder, we are ready to tackle the intellectual component of mental preparation: understanding how parents and teachers can nurture existing capacities in children to love, play, and create, and developing a working knowledge of vital relationships between brain, mind, body, and the pursuit of pleasure.

Optimal living is predicated on being able to integrate positive attitudes, creative proclivities, and well-formed values throughout the lifespan. What better place to begin our discussion of individual pathways to pleasure than childhood itself? Youth possess all the necessary "equipment" for a successful voyage of self-discovery: love, curiosity, and openness, permitting exquisite adaptation to an infinite variety of objects, people, and places. By understanding the basis for a positive childhood, we rise to the dual challenge of providing the best climate for our own progeny while helping to create a livable, survivable, humane world for posterity. Chapter 2: Nurturing the Healthy Child considers the nature of childhood and adolescent development. To a great extent, the process of self-discovery and the ability to feel naturally high depend on our sense of what we should provide for children. Equally significant is the fact that adult pleasure, in its most eloquent form, depends on our ability to recapture the spontaneity and unspoiled sense of beauty, wonder, and caring that flows from the creative spirit of childhood.

If we accept the notion that well-being depends, at least to some extent, on optimal brain functioning, then it behooves us to develop a basic understanding of the workings of that magnificent organ dubbed by Shakespeare as "the soul's frail dwelling place." In addition to its many other complex functions, the brain is also a molecular storehouse on which we can call to achieve pleasure. In 1974, J. Hughes and H. W. Kosterlitz discovered morphinelike compounds—endorphins—that exist naturally in the human brain, providing a biochemical foundation for the phenomenon of drug-free euphoria. The realization that the central nervous system can produce its own narcotics has since evolved into a reexamination of the fundamental causes of human behavior. In the past two decades, thousands of scientific treatises have explored relationships between thoughts, feelings, behavior, and brain chemistry.

One of the most intriguing aspects of the brain's "wiring" has to do with its limitations. As Sidney Cohen, author of *The Chemical Brain,* points out, "Brain circuitry permits momentary ecstasy or prolonged pleasure. Apparently, sustained ecstasy is neurophysiologically impossible." The earth-shattering "peak experience" drug users are seeking is, by its nature, fleeting; but that doesn't mean one can't develop the ability to engage in "prolonged pleasure" without the fireworks (or the damaging effects) of drug use. The choice between natural highs and artificial ones is actually a choice between two different kinds of brain functions, only one of which is truly sustainable over a lifetime.

Everyone can engage in activities that alter the brain's neurotransmission to produce "healthy intoxications." Heightened states of excitement, comfort, and increased self-awareness can all be accessed through certain forms of exercise, meditation, and other simple techniques. These experiences may seem tame, at first, compared to the use of potent drugs; the adjustment is not unlike weaning yourself from a diet loaded with salt and sugar in order to discern what food *really* tastes like. Still, people who understand how these states can be achieved without drugs are less likely to accept some of the traditional rationalizations about drug use (e.g., "LSD brings you closer to God," "Cocaine makes you a better lover").

Yet the process of pleasure isn't simply a matter of choice between a sustainable, beneficial altering of mood (natural highs) and a sudden, transient blast to the stratosphere (drugs). There is a psychological dimension to the kind of ecstasy we crave. Voluntary courtship of any drug or activity depends on how well it "fits" with one's usual style of coping. The drug of choice is actually a pharmacological defense mechanism; it bolsters already established patterns for managing psychological threat. People become addicted not to drugs or mood-altering behaviors as such, but to the sensations of pleasure that can be achieved through them. We repeatedly rely on three distinct types of experience to achieve feelings of well-being: *relaxation, excitement,* and *fantasy.* These three modes of pleasure are the underpinnings of human compulsion. As they say in show business, "You've gotta feed 'em, shock 'em, or amuse 'em."

Those who become excessively reliant on relaxation may gorge themselves with food, overindulge in watching TV, or use depressant drugs. They may partake in some or all of these activities simultaneously. Pleasure-seekers of this kind seek to reduce discomfort, which may originate from external events or internal conflict. They compulsively search for tranquillity, often to maintain control over their own hostility. When the universe is calm, there is less likelihood that they will lose composure and plunge into an uncontrolled fit of rage. As far as the brain is concerned, the chemical "payoff" for ritualized repose is like the effect of a sedative drug: TV addicts, for example, are tranquilizing themselves with visual Valium.

In sharp contrast, the compulsive thrill-seeker maintains a posture of active confrontation toward a world perceived as hostile and threatening. "Arousal" types tend to compensate for deep-seated feelings of inferiority through repeated attempts to demonstrate physical prowess or intellectual ability. They are usually extroverts, given to boasting about their sexual conquests, artistic talent, or mental agility. They tend to conceal their insecurities behind an overinflated sense of self-worth. Their energetic facade may be temporarily contrived through stimulant drugs and unnerving behavior. The sky diver's adrenaline rush is remarkably similar to the short, exhilarating jolt from a line of cocaine. Excessive risk-takers often mix danger with drugs.

Those compelled by fantasy enjoy activation of the right hemisphere of their cerebral cortex, using mental imagery to transport themselves into a state of either arousal or relaxation. T. S. Eliot once said, "To look into the heart is not enough. . . . One must also look into the cerebral cortex." His exhilarating passage "Hysteria" illustrates how provocative mental imagery can trigger a frenetic physical state:

> As she laughed I was aware of becoming involved in her laughter and being part of it, until her teeth were only accidental stars with a talent for squad-drill. I was drawn in by short gasps, inhaled at each momentary recovery, lost finally in the dark caverns of her throat, bruised by the ripple of unseen muscles. An elderly waiter with trembling hands was hurriedly spreading a pink and white checked cloth over the rusty green iron table, saying: "If the lady and gentleman wish to take their tea in the garden, if the lady and gentleman wish to take their tea in the garden. . . . " I decided that if the shaking of her breasts could be stopped, some of the fragments of the afternoon might be collected, and I concentrated my attention with careful subtlety to this end.

Those who court fantasy to excess may become lost in images and thoughts. There may be preoccupation with cosmic unity or spiritual oneness. Fantasy addicts maintain a special reverence for subtle nuances in interpersonal communication and are prone to find special meaning in accidental occurrences. Marijuana and hallucinogens such as LSD, psilocybin, and peyote are highly prized vehicles for imaginative transport.

The particular agents we select for relaxation, arousal, or fantasy escapes are determined, to some degree, by powerful social influences—everything from the kind of upbringing we had to the sort of technology available to us and the kinds of media images we are exposed to every day. Early predilections toward compulsive pleasure-seeking behavior may be inherited or learned from those around us—an alcoholic parent, a promiscuous relative, a neighbor who gambles. Preliminary patterns are then channeled by family and society into an array of potentially deviant careers, organized around drink, money, sex, calories, or whatever. We may find our means of escape in a particular drug or a particular outlet for compulsive behavior, such as public lotteries, telephone escort services, strip parlors and video arcades, or all-you-can-eat buffets. Whatever the medium, excessive reliance on activities that trigger sensations of arousal, relaxation, or fantasy is the basis for addictive behavior. In each case, an external prop is used to bring about a desired change in brain chemistry, until we come to rely on that prop in order to feel good.

Breaking the cycle of harmful pleasure-seeking doesn't mean denying a person's need to feel good. The objective of natural highs is to develop healthy means of arousal, relaxation, and fantasy, activities that "fit" individual circumstances and enhance a person's participation in everyday living, rather than offering a brief (and possibly one-way) trip to oblivion. By comprehending the biological, psychological, and social basis for pleasure-seeking—constructive or destructive—parents, educators, and community mentors can nurture healthy children who will later become healthy adults. Those prone to arousal can engage in exciting or challenging activities at each stage of development: gymnastics during childhood, competitive sports during adolescence, and so-called thrill sports or speculative business dealings during adulthood. These individuals can responsibly increase their rate of neurotransmission, thereby achieving an elevated level of mental alertness. Similarly, relaxation- or comfort-prone people can engage in desirable activities that decrease neuronal activity (reading, going to movies, or meditating) to achieve their coveted mental state. For those who thrive on imagination, fantasy escapades triggered by art, music, stories, myths, fairy tales, and legends may prove truly beneficial.

Optimal health and well-being, of course, derive from an ideal balance of novel and stimulating activity, comfort and creative imagination. People who realize their potential seem to enjoy nearly equal investments of energy in their work, love, and play. Their spirituality is reflected by an ability to integrate a profound sense of moral responsibility with everyday behaviors. If drug prevention efforts in the schools have been less than successful, it may be because the present system doesn't sufficiently involve the family and the community in fostering strong social values. It is, after all, much easier to push information or emotionally charged imagery ("This is your brain on drugs") than values. Yet imagine what the effect might be if, in addition to the Pledge of Allegiance, schoolchildren started their day by reciting this passage by Ralph Waldo Emerson:

To laugh often and much;
To win the respect of intelligent people and
affection of children;
To earn the appreciation of honest critics and
endure the betrayal of false friends;
To appreciate beauty;
To find the best in others;
To leave the world a bit better, whether by a healthy
child, a garden patch or a redeemed social
condition;
To know even one life has breathed easier
because you have lived.
This is to have succeeded.

A positive outlook and a grasp of the fundamentals of brain chemistry can certainly provide the mental preparation for natural highs. But taking the plunge involves developing the emotional and behavioral competencies to "laugh often and much," to appreciate beauty, and, finally, to succeed.

Skill Development

"Natural highs" skills are actually new ways of coping. Acquiring them is a matter of first becoming more at ease with yourself and your relationships with others, and then identifying and developing individual talents and abilities that yield healthy pleasures. The process can be divided into four stages: relaxing, setting healthy boundaries, seeking a meaningful engagement of talents, and cultivating body awareness.

Relaxing

Relaxation is the gateway to natural highs. Enjoyment of healthy pleasures is impossible as long as we are tense, restless, or devoured by anxiety. Some people attempt to deal with such feelings through intensive self-sedation, such as the television "addicts" described above, but true relaxation is neither compulsive nor stultifying. Rather, it is a physiological bridge to that elusive state we sometimes refer to as "peace of mind."

Ever since the Beatles helped popularize transcendental meditation, Western culture has embarked on a tentative exploration of a multitude of widely available, little-understood, and underutilized self-soothing techniques. Given the amount of research that's been done on the benefits of meditation and other quick-and-easy means to relaxation, it's surprising that these techniques are still underutilized by most stress-riddled Americans. Our journey begins at home, learning to focus our thoughts and to become more comfortable by learning to relax. Joan Borysenko, author of *Minding the Body, Mending the Mind*, put it best when she said, "All the experiences in life are like zeros in a long number. They are meaningless without a digit in front of them. That digit is peace of mind."

Setting Healthy Boundaries

To develop the competence and confidence to manage our lives effectively, we need to set what psychologists call healthy boundaries. That means recognizing and defining your independent, separate identity, without becoming confused by the whims, needs, and demands of others.

The lack of such boundaries contributes to the emotional chaos found in alcoholic, abusive, or otherwise dysfunctional families. Parents whose parenting skills are overwhelmed by their own emotional problems manage to "pass on" aspects of their inappropriate behavior to their children, who tend to be fast learners. When a child combines his or her natural assertiveness, necessary for survival, with an overabundance of parental anger, the result is a personality confounded by rage. Similarly, when we assimilate parental pain, in addition to our own, the result is depression. Childhood fear combined with overwhelming parental anxiety equals panic; and perhaps most troubling of all, the emotion of shame—which is tormenting to children of alcoholic and other mentally disordered parents—plus existing parental baggage equals humiliation.

Remember Mary Barnes's reference to a "bottomless hole inside me," which she thought could be "filled" only with drugs? Without a clear sense of emotional or spiritual boundaries, we can easily go astray trying to fill that hole. Carl Jung once remarked, "The thirst for alcohol on a lower level can be compared to men and women's thirst for wholeness, union and completeness." In other words, drug and alcohol abuse are compensatory for our failing ability to reach peak or spiritual experiences.

In 1931, Roland H.—one of the cofounders of Alcoholics Anonymous—had a particularly enlightening conversation with Jung. Roland H. came to the famed psychiatrist because of his drinking problem; Jung frankly told him that he was a hopeless case, that the available medical or psychiatric treatments were inadequate. When he then asked if there was any other hope, Jung advised him that there might be, provided he could become the subject of a spiritual or religious experience. He did just that, finding deliverance in what AA literature refers to as belief in "a higher power." Ironically, Roland H.'s recovery has spawned a kind of quasi-religious movement. Today there are more than 8,000 AA groups worldwide, and more than 15 million Americans participate in self-help groups styled on the AA twelve-step philosophy, groups ranging from Sexaholics Anonymous to Fundamentalists Anonymous. A Newsweek journalist described this situation thus:

All of a sudden, people are pouring back into the churches and synagogues with a fervor that hasn't been seen since the '50s. It appears that a great religious revival is sweeping the land—until you examine the situation a little more closely. Then you will notice the biggest crowds today often arrive in midweek, and instead of filing into the pews these people head for the basement, where they immediately sit down and begin talking about their deepest secrets, darkest fears and strangest cravings.

Alcoholics? Third door to the right. Sex addicts? They meet on Tuesday. Overweight men who have a problem with compulsive shopping? Pull up a folding chair, buddy, you're in the right place.

Many of us encounter a spiritual gap in our experience, a discontinuity between the intuitive, instinctual nature of humankind and the spiritual or godlike qualities within us all.

Within me are the dark immemorial forces of the Evil One, human and pre-human; Within me too are the luminous forces, human and pre-human, of God—and my soul is the arena where these two armies have clashed and met.

—N. Kazantzakis

The alcoholic or drug abuser, who as much as anyone else may be described as "simply human," experiences this conflict even more intensely. In the words of Abraham Lincoln (1842),

> In my judgment, such of us as have never fallen victims, have been spared more from the absence of appetite, than from any mental or moral superiority over those who have. Indeed, I believe if we take habitual drunkards as a class, their heads and their hearts would bear an advantageous comparison with those of any other class.

From a spiritual perspective, an addict is a person who is other worldly directed, however misguided in the management of this calling. Substances are used to compensate, to fill the void, the "hole in the soul." Hallucinogens are ingested by some to promote the illusion of spirituality. Alcohol may provide entrance to the world of instincts and sensuality.

Must one come to a religious awakening before being released from a compulsive pleasure-seeking orientation? Probably not. True, religious symbols—"higher powers"—have been effective in removing addicts from their misguided or clumsy attempts to achieve the ecstasy of wholeness. When a person incorporates a religious figure such as Buddha or Christ, the meaning of life changes dramatically. But symbols of unity and transcendence are also basic to music, poetry, literature, and art. The depth and fluidity of one's life can also be enhanced by secular symbols that represent nature, aesthetics, and neighborly love.

There is a broad range of symbolic devices for self-realization and completeness. Depending on one's personal belief system and ability to incorporate the life of the spirit with the workings of the brain, healthy mood-altering experiences can become opportunities to achieve particularly intense and meaningful states of altered consciousness. In any case, the increased sense of self-contained pleasure and accomplishment one can acquire through natural highs can keep us "on track" in the effort to establish healthy boundaries.

Seeking a Meaningful Engagement of Talents

One of the recurrent themes of drug prevention programs in the schools is the threat of wasted potential. "If you take drugs," warns the visiting celebrity athlete (or scholar or ballerina), "you'll never be a famous athlete [scholar, ballerina] like me!"

Well intentioned as these testimonials are, they often fall on deaf ears. Sooner or later, young people discover that there *are* famous athletes, performers, and even educators who take drugs (never mind that the drugs may end their careers). And most adolescents have difficulty subscribing to the notion of delayed gratification—years of hard work and study in order to profit somewhere down the line. They want to feel good *now*—and let's face it, as far as brain chemistry is concerned, drugs generally pack a short-term wallop well beyond anything natural highs can offer. As one colleague of ours quipped recently, playing devil's advocate, "Anyone who calls it a runner's high obviously never took any real drugs."

Still, it would be foolish to try to come up with a jolt-for-jolt substitute for drug use. Viable alternatives to drugs and alcohol can be found only through an individualized program designed to develop one's potential skills and talents; the process is vital not only in drug prevention and education but in recovery. When former drug users who have discovered "improved" methods of altering consciousness are interviewed, a common thread in their stories of recovery is their success at achieving a "meaningful engagement of talents"—identifying and nurturing their secret "gift" for art, athletics, technology, handicrafts, business, or whatever. Participating in activities that interest you, that you excel at, and that are productive not only increases your experience of the natural highs associated with those activities (short-term gratification), but proves to be a long-term investment in self-esteem.

How do we encourage this stirring of dormant potential, particularly for the nearly 25 percent of the population that struggles with addictive/compulsive behavior, the millions of Americans who perceive themselves as inept vis-à-vis contemporary society? One way is to rethink our notions of excellence, so that we may aggressively seek out talent in young people and fan its spark. There is growing evidence that our society's traditional definition of intelligence has systematically deprived thousands of students of the opportunity to excel. Harvard psychologist Howard Gardner, among others, has attacked IQ tests as being far too limited in their ability to measure the aptitude of diverse racial and ethnic groups: "They sample only a tiny firmament of human abilities, and we're somehow making the IQ score equal to all intelligence."

In his book *Frames of Mind,* Gardner suggests that large-scale recognition of "multiple intelligences" will enable educators to transcend their customary reliance on verbal and mathematical abilities in evaluating students' intelligence and potential, often to the exclusion of other factors. Table 1.1 shows the multiple intelligences that have been described by Gardner and his associates. Collectively, they offer a direct challenge to parochial attitudes about what constitutes adaptive strength and general problem-solving skills.

TABLE 1.1
Seven Ways to Be Bright

Linguistic
Language skills include a sensitivity to the subtle shades of the meanings of words.

Logical—Mathematical
Both critics and supporters acknowledge that IQ tests measure this ability well.

Musical
Like language, music is an expression medium—and this talent flourishes in prodigies.

Spacial
Sculptors and painters are able accurately to perceive, manipulate, and re-create forms.

Bodily—Kinesthetic
At the core of this kink of intelligence are body control and skilled handling of objects.

Interpersonal
Skill in reading the moods and intentions of others is displayed by politicians, among others.

Intrapersonal
The key is understanding one's own feelings—and using that insight to guide behavior.

Source: U.S. News & World Report, November, 1987, p. 53

In several well-designed programs throughout the United States, select students are beginning to reap the benefits of Gardner's approach. The Educational Testing Service in Princeton, New Jersey, has supported a pilot program in Pittsburgh schools to evaluate artistic abilities. In Indianapolis, an elementary school has initiated the development of a curriculum in all seven intelligence areas. Project Spectrum, which Gardner designed with Tufts University psychologist David Feldman, helps parents and teachers identify children's strengths and interests at a young age.

Chapter 4: Using Your Inner Resources explores other approaches to a meaningful engagement of talents. Not surprisingly, "talent-scouting" within yourself often requires you to see yourself and your surroundings in a new light—perhaps "to see the world anew each day." One of us (Milkman) recently had just such an eye-opening experience, one suggesting that the younger the subject, the easier this process can be:

> Last night, my wife, Meredith, took me aside and said, "Look at this sculpture." Offhandedly, without much consideration, I replied, "Yes, it's pretty." She said, "You're not even listening." Just then, I realized that Merry was requesting a perceptual shift. Rather than mere lip service, she wanted me to really look. I knew exactly what she meant—the *artist's eye*. Suddenly, I could perceive the glistening water, magnificent luminosity, subtle differences in shading, razor-sharp angles, glowing effervescence. The "water sculpture" transformed from a bland, nondescript, rather colorless form to a highly differentiated objet d'art. I became conscious of patterns and shapes, glistening refractions of light. Then I invited Tasha, our daughter, who was then two years old, to share in the experience. She giggled with joy as she touched the water cascading down the magical sculpture. Already, she was well acquainted with the artist's eye.

Cultivating Body Awareness

One of the strongest weapons in our arsenal against drugs is a commonsense approach to exercise and nutrition. Students of brain chemistry know there is more than a grain of truth in the biblical dictum "The body is the temple of the soul." A more modern (and more prosaic) rendering might be this: exercise and nutrition are the physical keys to mood regulation and feelings of well-being.

That vigorous exercise can alter mood has been known for ages, but the phenomenon has been studied scientifically only for the past thirty years. More recently, the popular press has taken up the banner of exercise as a cure-all for depression, anxiety, fatigue, insomnia, stress, and other psychological illnesses. We have been bombarded with slick articles touting the benefits of "runner's high," "exercise euphoria," "running away from depression," and other often unsubstantiated claims.

While exercise isn't an all-purpose panacea, the "Exercise! Not the couch!" advocates did receive a tremendous boost with the 1974 discovery of endorphins, the body's internal opiates. Subsequent studies have shown that exercise increases the level of endorphins in blood plasma. While there is some concern that endorphins produced in the plasma may not cross into the brain, the mood-altering effects of vigorous exercise have been well documented. A report issued following a 1984 conference at the National Institute of Mental Health listed several direct benefits of exercise on mood alteration and mental health in general. Exercise, which leads to physical fitness and builds self-esteem, is an excellent way to achieve a natural high.

What is less well known is that changes in diet can have an effect on brain chemistry similar to (though usually less dramatic than) that of a graduated program of exercise. The prevalent attitude for many years was that, because of the blood-brain barrier, the brain was generally impervious to assaults from junk food and other atrocious comestibles. Although a steady diet of Twinkies and Ho-Hos may cause our bodies to disintegrate into mush, we expected that our brains would continue to function "normally."

This attitude persisted despite considerable folklore extolling the virtues of certain foods in altering moods or enhancing mental ability. For example, our grandmothers told us that a snack of milk and cookies before bedtime would help us to relax and fall asleep. We ate fish for "brainpower" and oysters for sexual potency.

Today, with our knowledge of brain chemistry, we are beginning to develop a clearer sense of the links between diet and brain function. We know, for example, that in order for the brain to function normally, there must be a relatively constant level of molecules called neurotransmitters. These molecules carry information from one cell to the next. We also know that certain amino acids present in our diet have the ability to go from the blood to the brain, where they are converted into neurotransmitters, such as serotonin, dopamine, and norepinephrine.

A major breakthrough in our understanding of the relationship between diet and mood came in 1974, when J. D. Fernstrom and R. J. Wurtman published their research establishing that the amino acid tryptophan, when ingested, increased the level of serotonin in the brains of laboratory rats. Tryptophan is found in a number of foods, including milk. In addition, Fernstrom and Wurtman showed that a diet high in carbohydrates also increased the level of serotonin in the brain. Since serotonin has been associated with relaxation and sleep, it turns out that Grandma was right after all—a snack of milk and cookies won't knock you out like sodium pentothal, but it just might hasten the onset of sleep.

We also know that the excitatory neurotransmitters responsible for alertness and wakefulness are produced from the amino acid tyrosine, which is found in animal protein. Other studies have traced the chemical basis for the much-touted soothing or stimulating effects of various herb and plant extracts that may be as potent mood-changers as sugar or caffeine, without the detrimental effects of those more prevalent additives. Equipped with this kind of information, we should be able to exert some control over our moods by the food we eat. For example, if we want to remain alert in the afternoon, it would be wise to eat a lunch rich in protein and skip the carbohydrates. On the other hand, cookies and milk can be an excellent sedative. We might be led to conclude that

Bread is for going to bed;
Steak is for staying awake.

Many people regard working out and eating right in rather dreary terms, as things they "should" be doing in order to ward off fat, evade early mortality, and keep up with all the fitness fanatics they see torturing themselves in the public parks and private health clubs. Exercise and nutrition are seen as "maintenance programs" or as a kind of penance for bad behavior, rather than as a benefit in themselves—except, perhaps, to those fanatics who have made a formidable cult out of calories saved or burned. Yet there is another way to look at the issue: exercise and nutrition have an essential, dramatic, and positive role in the pursuit of healthy pleasures. Taking charge of pleasure means taking charge of your body *and* your brain chemistry. Educating yourself on the effects that various foods and physical activities have on your mood and acting on that information in a sensible, appropriate way will certainly increase your ability to achieve natural highs.

Implementation

Valuable as the "natural highs" skills are to the pursuit of pleasure, they are not ends in themselves. In our seminars, we have always emphasized that the true enjoyment of these activities is not, in essence, selfish hedonism; rather, it depends on the integration of these skills in a large social context. The concept of natural highs makes little or no sense without the nurturing and support of human relatedness. People can swim, jump, row, dance, sing, finger-paint, or stand on their heads without feeling any sense of fulfillment. Proficiency cannot be equated with happiness.

One way that the experience of natural highs becomes infused with greater meaning—that is, meaning *beyond* the immediate sensation of personal pleasure—is by incorporating these activities in ritualized forms that help to define one's role and responsibilities in society. Our culture has lost or abandoned many of its traditional ceremonies for expressing crucial transitions in our lives. For example, religious rituals marking the passage to adulthood, such as the Catholic Confirmation or the Jewish Bar Mitzvah, have become, for many of us, dead forms, artifacts from another era. Yet the need for rites of passage and initiation remains; for many youngsters, Club MTV and teenage gangs have replaced the esprit de corps of team sports and social groups.

We examine ways to develop new "ceremonies of transition" in Chapter 8: Celebrating Life. Ideally, such rituals become a springboard for individuals to develop the kinds of social skills that will serve them well throughout their adult lives, nurturing a network of caring relationships that supports and enhances the experience of healthy pleasures.

Indeed, human connectedness—so difficult to measure—has recently been documented as the foundation for health and well-being. In the April 1989 issue of *Scientific American,* Emmy Werner published the findings of her thirty-year study, findings that underscore the vital importance of adult nurturing. In 1955, all 698 children who were born on the Hawaiian island of Kauai participated in Werner's study, which followed their development at one, two, ten, eighteen, thirty-one, or thirty-two years of age. While 422 were judged to have a supportive environment, 201 were considered at risk for developing some form of emotional or behavioral disorder later in life. These vulnerable youth had four of the following risk factors prior to their second birthday: perinatal stress, chronic poverty, parents' education level less than the eighth grade, family discord, divorce. They constituted 30 percent of the surviving children on the island. Two-thirds of these children (129 in all) did develop serious learning or behavioral problems by age ten or had delinquency records, mental health problems, or pregnancies by the time they were eighteen.

More important, one out of three did not! Seventy-two of these high-risk children grew into competent young adults who loved, worked, and played well. The research team was able to identify a number of factors that seemed to protect vulnerable children from poor adjustment. Their temperaments were characterized by high activity, low excitability and distress, and high sociability.

Their social circumstances were perhaps even more revealing. Kids who remained healthy had four or fewer children in their immediate family. There were at least two years between the birth of siblings. The at-risk children who succeeded had emotional support outside of their immediate family. They participated in extracurricular activities and had formed a close bond with one or more caretakers during the first years of life. Of paramount importance was the establishment of at least one genuine caring relationship. Werner found that "the resilient children in [her] study had at least one person in their lives who accepted them unconditionally regardless of temperamental idiosyncrasies or physical or mental handicaps." Her most significant finding is that

> all children can be helped to become more resilient if adults in their lives encourage independence, teach them appropriate communication and self-help skills and model, as well as reward, acts of helpfulness and caring.

The importance of a creative and caring environment for high-risk children has also received increasing scrutiny—and media coverage—on the mainland. An episode of "Sixty Minutes" featured Tom Pilecki, a former Franciscan who has turned St. Augustine's Church, located in the impoverished Morrisania section of the South Bronx in New York City, into a school for the arts. Each student learns two musical instruments and studies ballet and modern dance. Business courses emphasize pride in one's job, leading to feelings of dignity and self-worth. Humanities courses focus on the historical relationship between the aristocracy and the working class. In a short time, the enrollment at the school soared to more than 300, with nearly every student reading at grade level or higher.

The project's success is attributed to the conscious choice that parents and children make to participate in the stimulating learning atmosphere, where Shakespeare is taught with enthusiasm, where candy and junk food are forbidden, and where self-respect, appreciation for one another, and pride in what the children have mastered are all valued. The staff of St. Augustine's is inspired by the knowledge that, as Pilecki puts it, "We stand a chance of giving the kids a real sense of what can be. It doesn't have to be what's out on the street; . . . it can be something very different."

". . . a real sense of what can be." How we deal with life's challenges, our ways of coping with pleasure and pain, is inextricably bound up with family and social relationships, our own sense of ourselves and our abilities, and our mastery of our own bodies and minds.

All of us possess the amazing ability to manufacture neurochemicals that change our moods. We can learn to use our brain chemistry to feel good naturally through song and dance and laughter, through loving ourselves and the people around us. These ideals, self-evident as they may be, are difficult to attain. The remainder of this book is designed to help us get there.

Mental Preparation

2

Nurturing the Healthy Child

What Shall We Give the Children?

It seems certain that they will travel roads we never thought of, navigate strange seas, cross unimagined boundaries and glimpse horizons beyond our power to visualize. What can we give them to take along? For the wild shores Beyond, no toy or bauble will do. It must be something more, constructed of stouter fabric discovered among the cluttered aisles and tinseled bargain counters of experience, winnowed from what little we have learned. It must be devised out of responsibility and profound caring, a homemade present of selfless love. Everything changes but the landscape of the heart.

What shall we give the children?

Attention, for one day it will be too late.

A sense of value, the inalienable place of the individual in the scheme of things, with all that accrues to the individual—self-reliance, courage, conviction, self-respect and respect for others.

A sense of humor. Laughter leavens life.

The meaning of discipline. If we falter at discipline, life will do it for us.

The will to work. Satisfying work is the lasting you.

The talent for sharing, for it is not so much what we give as what we share.

The love of justice. Justice is the bulwark against violence and oppression and the repository of human dignity.

The passion for truth, founded on precept and example. Truth is the beginning of every good thing.

The power of faith, engendered in mutual trust. Life without faith is a dismal dead-end street.

The beacon of hope, which lights all darkness.

The knowledge of being loved beyond demand or reciprocity, praise or blame, for those so loved are never lost.

What shall we give the children?

*The open sky, the brown earth, the hefty tree, the golden sand, the blue
    water, the stars in their courses and the awareness of these. Bird song,
    butterflies, clouds and rainbows. Sunlight, moonlight, firelight.*
*A large hand reaching down for a small hand, impromptu praise, an
    unexpected kiss, a straight answer.*
The glisten of enthusiasm and a sense of wonder.
Long days to be merry in and nights without fear.
The memory of a good home.

—*Anonymous*

No challenge in life, it seems, generates so much hope and anxiety,
such wild idealism and burdensome sense of responsibility, as parenthood. Every new parent yearns to provide his or her child with
boundless love and happiness, a strong sense of values and self-
worth, a vast array of material comforts—in short, the perfect
"good home." Of course, perfection in childrearing tends to elude
even the most enthusiastic parent, but the desire to nurture, to try to
shape a healthy environment for our children, is one of the driving
forces of human existence.

Before embarking on a detailed discussion of brain chemistry
(Chapter 3), it's helpful to consider a few fundamental aspects of the
process of child and adolescent development. So much of who we
are was shaped by choices made years ago by our own parents or
guardians, just as so much of who our children will be is being
shaped by choices we make today. At this time in human history, we
find it particularly meaningful to consider the lives of people who
are a generation or two down the road. The distinct challenge of our
time is to create a livable, survivable, humane world for posterity.
Some may ask, "Why should I care about people I will never know
and see? What did the future ever do for me?" But posterity can do
something for all of us. We shall not live to see many of our most
cherished hopes and values come to pass. Therefore, the dream of
fulfilling human potential—of optimal living through natural
highs—is to some extent lodged in others at a later time. Indeed,
some of the most pleasurable feelings of delight and celebration,
courage and hope, are bound to people, places, and events not yet
seen.

No one can make the "right" choice all the time; indeed, in many
instances there may be no right or wrong about it. Yet the biochem-

ical and psychological processes involved in our journey from infant to adult hold important clues for us. They tell us how certain experiences influence and even define our mode of pleasure-seeking; they also provide us with a road map of sorts that tells us how to go about creating a healthy, nurturing environment for ourselves and our children.

Earlier we noted that the mental preparation for learning to cultivate creative promise, to take charge of pleasure, begins with a shift in attitude about pleasure itself—a revival of the childlike sense of wonder, combined with a deeper understanding of the way the brain works. What better way to begin, then, than to try once more to see the world through the eyes of a child?

Coming into the World

Magnea Jonsdottir, Icelander, age thirty-nine, and John Hopkins, American, age thirty-three, are an unmarried couple who reside in Reykjavik, Iceland. They recently learned that Magnea is pregnant. Like most expectant parents, they are discovering that the prospect of welcoming their first child into the world has stirred a wide range of hopes and fears, plans and dreams.

Magnea: When I first found out, I didn't really want to take it in. I doubted the test. I began to feel strange—simultaneous planning, confusion, and getting acquainted with the notion that there was a new life inside me.

But the real feeling would come later the same day. I had an appointment with my best girlfriend. I was waiting to tell her and finally I did. Suddenly, we both broke out in laughter. Just then was the first time I felt that something real was happening. . . . I became anxious, too.

I waited three weeks to see John, to tell him the news in person.

John: It was a rush like the ground dropped away from my feet—whoosh—butterflies and all that stuff. I was a little shaky, I guess. I began to wonder how this would affect my life.

Not surprisingly, Magnea and John expect that many of their activities over the next few months will revolve around the pregnancy. Magnea vows to have "a healthy life—good food, fresh air, and movement." They are even planning a ritual celebration of sorts.

Magnea: I will have to train myself to get in contact with that little human being that I don't yet feel by making physical contact with my belly, like saying [gently placing her palm on her abdomen], "Good morning."

I would like to involve my partner actively in the pregnancy by asking him to go on a journey with me: my imaginative journey.

John: We'll do a ceremony at a holy place in the Mohave Desert. I guess you'd call it a blessing or a welcoming ceremony. I don't choreograph, but I've been there several times. . . . It's a power point, an energy source, a magic place.

Magnea: I will have a drum. I've inherited this old coat from my aunt. It's getting old and broken, and I need to say goodbye to it, so we decided to bury the coat as part of the ceremony.

Magnea and John have given a great deal of thought to what will happen once the baby is born.

Magnea: I will encourage intimate contact—the full expression of emotions within the family. I will give the child a lot of care; to let the child feel that it is really cared for is very important. I will provide a deep sense of security by being around, . . . hearing all the little sounds, seeing all the little signals, and responding to them.

We'll play outdoors a lot and, when the baby is bigger, draw, paint, develop hobbies, and tell stories.

John: I'll try not to control or restrict the child, striving for some balance in structured freedom. I'm an idealist, so I would like to create an awareness of truth in terms of the natural and spiritual world. I want our child to see through the falseness of culture and society and look for true wisdom.

I want to involve the child in my own explorations of life and spirit; physical process and movement; sensory action; looking at the world.

Magnea: In terms of values, equality is very important—that everybody is equal. I will teach respect and love for animals and nature. Honesty and modesty; being a social person but also to be a strong individual who asserts his or her rights. . . . It has something to do with self-confidence.

John: I would like to help this child to appreciate the weakness of the dominant morality of this age, the basic profanity of cultural values. I want to cultivate a level of independence that allows for true freethinking, to cultivate an awareness of the limitations of material pursuits. Instead of thinking about all the things that I have the right to get from life, I would promote the idea that one has obligations for others, rather than rights to be claimed from them. This is a personal philosophy that may be difficult to implement, given the prevailing cultural milieu.

Magnea: Right now, I'm starting to feel happiness about some of the things that are growing between the two of us. A change of the relationship, I'm not sure how. I feel more respect, more closeness, and maybe something that has not come yet, . . . but it's starting to develop within me— a letting go of the self-centeredness—I'm looking forward to this.

The Developing Brain

While John and Magnea may sound slightly more idealistic than some parents, the kinds of concerns they voice—concerns about their child's physical and emotional welfare, the values and behavior they would like to encourage—are fairly typical. Much of what they have to say about their plans, such as Magnea's desire to lead a healthy life ("good food, fresh air, exercise, and movement"), may strike the reader as nothing more than simple common sense. But the sort of childrearing choices that parents make take on an added significance in light of what we now know about how the brain develops in the first weeks and months of life.

We know, for example, that within hours of fertilization, the egg begins to divide again and again, producing trillions of cells, each capable of specialized tasks. Hidden within each cell is a chemical blueprint that controls what it will become—muscles, bones, tissue, vital organs, and the nervous system. One group of cells will become the brain, a giant electrochemical computer, eventually capable of comprehending symbols, language, and abstract concepts such as freedom and honesty. In the first few weeks, a tube begins to form, which is the first step in the development of the brain. As the tube matures, a layer of cells appears, soon to become neurons, which form the basis for all brain activities.

Magnea's concern for the baby in utero is well founded. A critical period for neuronal development occurs between eight and sixteen weeks following conception. During this time, the rudimentary brain begins to differentiate into glial cells and neurons. By the eighth week, glial cells—structural girders of the brain—begin to send out fibers toward the brain's information-processing components, neurons. The glial cells nourish the neurons and help them migrate to their destinations. The genetically choreographed dance between neurons and glial cells, culminating in billions of synaptic communities, is perhaps the most vital part of human growth and development.

The harmony of natural migration may, however, be interrupted by environmental insult. Alcohol, for example, causes neurons to grow past their destinations. The resultant Fetal Alcohol Syndrome (FAS) and, to a lesser degree, Fetal Alcohol Effects (FAE) reflect varying degrees of physical deformity, mental retardation, and emotional and behavioral disorders. Although the incidence of Fetal Drug Syndrome (FDS) is also being studied, specific drug effects are difficult to identify. Low birthweight has been associated with cigarette smoking and cocaine use, but it is difficult to determine how often these drugs were used in combination with each other and/or with alcohol.

While researchers are still grappling with the wide array of effects on the fetus of parental drug abuse, proper prenatal care has evolved from a medical issue to a legal one. On July 13, 1989, Jennifer Johnson became the first woman in the United States to be convicted of delivering a controlled substance to a minor as a result of her drug use during pregnancy. Even though the Florida law under which she was tried states that it is a felony for an adult to deliver drugs to a minor, the question of a drug-using woman's responsibility to the unborn was deftly skirted. L. H. Glantz describes how the prosecution was able to successfully argue its case:

> Since as a legal matter the delivery under this law must be made to a person and fetuses are not deemed persons for this purpose, the prosecution argued that the delivery transpired in the 60 to 90 seconds when the baby was delivered but before the umbilical cord was cut. The prosecution argued that during this time an umbilical cord is "no different from a hypodermic needle, straw or other device that functions to introduce a substance into the body." Thus at the moment of giving birth, Ms. Johnson became a drug pusher and the umbilical cord became a piece of drug paraphernalia.

Unfortunately, drugs and alcohol are only the most immediate of a wide range of environmental hazards that can endanger the fetus. For example, even a relatively mild dose of radiation, such as that one might receive from a single Xray, can disrupt fetal brain development. Radioactivity affects neuronal migration in a manner similar to the way alcohol does. While alcohol causes neurons to continue growing past their destinations, radiation stops them short of their targets; in both bases, however, newly emerging cells are killed at a critical stage of brain development. Research conducted in the aftermath of the American nuclear attack on Hiroshima and Nagasaki indicates that the rate of mental retardation among fetuses exposed to radiation may be five times higher than it is in the general population. Given the potential for another Chernobyl-like meltdown, particularly among primitive and flawed nuclear reactors still operating in the former Soviet Union, is it any wonder the "no-nukes" movement seems to be heavily staffed with mothers and their small children?

Other teratogens (external factors that may interfere with the developing fetus) can be ingested through air, food, or water. Pesticides sprayed on vegetation and underground toxic wastes are suspected of causing miscarriages, stillbirths, and birth defects. Benzene found in cleaning fluids; carbon monoxide from cigarette smoke and automobile exhaust; carbon disulfide, hydrocarbons, lead, and mercury in food; and vinyl chloride, a compound used to make plastic, are common substances known to adversely affect the growing fetus. NutraSweet, a popular sugar substitute, is now under close scrutiny, too. Still, although potentially hazardous chemicals are constantly in our midst, damage is not inevitable. Human beings have tremendous resilience, and even when exposed to potential harm, most fetuses develop normally—3 to 6 percent of the babies born today are structurally impaired.

The best protection against problems during pregnancy is regular monitoring by a qualified obstetrician—and, of course, mindful avoidance of harmful substances. The latter point has become the urgent message of prenatal education in contemporary America, particularly those programs aimed at pregnant teenagers. Recently an unusual musical, *Don't Wait until You See Me,* debuted in Chicago high schools; the play, which dramatizes events in the womb of a fourteen-year-old girl, is designed to get other young expectant mothers thinking about their fetus's welfare. The basic plot is as follows:

> On the exact day that the teenage mother-to-be finally hears from the doctor that, in fact, she is pregnant, she assaults herself with cigarettes and alcohol, and seriously considers taking cocaine. Baby-in-the-womb is almost poisoned by pollution from the toxic indulgences. Although she refuses a suggested drink, she is informed that the decision, after all, is not hers. "If your mother drinks, you drink. . . . "
> The finale of the works occurs on the 61st day of pregnancy with the expectant mother and baby-to-be continuing the battle between positive and negative attractions.

After those first two critical months, fetal development begins to accelerate at an astonishing pace. When maturation is normal, the brain begins to stabilize by the eighteenth week. At twenty-one weeks, hearing begins to occur, and at twenty-six weeks, although the fetus lives in total darkness, the visual apparatus begins to function. Infants who are born three to four months prematurely are already capable of seeing, hearing, and surviving in an extrauterine environment.

Magnea's idea of making contact with the baby while it is still in the womb is clearly guided by intuitive acumen. The newborn shows a distinct preference for its own mother's voice over other female voices. In laboratory demonstrations, newborns will suck on a nipple longer when they hear a familiar voice. The baby's nursing response demonstrates that biology prepares the infant to respond to its mother while still in the womb—"Good morning," little Magnea or John.

Even though the neonate is prepared to survive in the flood of novel—sometimes painful—stimuli outside the womb, the developing brain remains vulnerable for some time after birth. Using animal models, scientists have determined that during the first year of life the brain assembles a neurological map of sounds, objects, and events in the outside world. The mouse, for example, has sixty-six whiskers, thirty-three on each side of its upper lip. The whiskers move in concert, navigating tactile space for the mouse as a blind person would use his or her cane. During the first days of life, a specific area of the brain becomes structurally "committed" to receiving sensory data from each whisker. If the whiskers are removed before the mouse is five days old, the whisker-sensitive area of the brain ceases to function. When, however, the whiskers are severed from the sixth day onward, the sensory map inside the mouse's brain remains unchanged—the brain has already declared its preference for this type of input, as it were. Through this process, which is similar to that which occurs in the human brain, neural functioning becomes more efficient; neurons that are not "committed" die off.

Researchers are still seeking to delineate and understand the process by which the brain commits itself to specific types of stimuli. For example, infants are born with the flexibility to learn any language. By the end of the first year of life, however, babies who are exposed to English can no longer discriminate some of the sounds from a different language, which has now become simply an alien or "foreign" group of sounds. But why does this happen at this particular stage of growth?

The implications of this kind of research for prospective parents are enormous. The developing brain receives "marching orders" not only from an inborn molecular guidance mechanism within the brain itself, but also from the outside environment. Consequently, the kind of attentive, warm, stimulating care that parenting gurus urge on us so that we might "bond" with our children—the kind of doting parenthood Magnea and John are looking forward to with such eagerness—turns out to be a good idea in terms of brain development, too. It promotes the child's active exploration of his or her surroundings, allowing the brain to optimize its continued growth and refinement.

But what happens to the child's mental growth if the environment does not provide stimulation and nurturing? A considerable body of evidence supports the notion that children who grow up "deprived"—as a result of poverty, malnutrition, neglect, abuse, and other factors—suffer a higher incidence of mental retardation and other neurological handicaps. Adherents of this view often cite research involving a comparison of animals reared in nonstimulative isolation with those raised in stimulating environments. Those living in comfortable surroundings have a higher ratio of differentiated (specialized functioning) to undifferentiated brain cells. Extrapolating from this finding, one can expect that an infant will fail to develop certain brain cell functions as a consequence of social deprivation.

For many of these children, school often comes too late. Before they cross their first schoolyard, considerable damage has already been done to their chances to "catch up." Yet there is also evidence that, in many cases, the neuronal deficit associated with early deprivation need not be permanent. Studies conducted since the 1940s of impoverished children suggest that infancy should be considered a "sensitive" rather than "critical" phase of development. And it's even possible for severely deprived babies to "catch up" under the right circumstances, although doing so apparently becomes more difficult after the second year of life.

Consider the fate of babies raised in Creche, a Lebanese institution, who showed signs of extreme retardation in motor and language development after they spent their first year basically languishing in their cribs. Many did not sit up until they were a year old or begin to walk until they were three or four; the average IQ for one- to six-year-olds was 53 (a normal IQ is 100). In 1956, when adoption became legal in Lebanon, many of these children found adoptive parents and secure homes. Those who left the institution before the age of two overcame their initial retardation and gained an average of more than 50 IQ points, achieving a score of about 100 within two years' time. In sharp contrast, later adoptees, although they showed some improvement in IQ, never fully recovered from their retardation.

We have moved from considering a critical in-womb phase of a few weeks to a sensitive period of development spanning the first two years of life. Some might argue that childrearing is a "sensitive" matter well into adolescence; but no matter what time frame is being considered, the commitment to nurture a child is a statement of profound optimism—a declaration of sorts that life is not only worth living but worth sharing and savoring. The process of sharing actually begins in the womb, of course, but it becomes a much more sophisticated business in the first days of life, as parents start to key themselves to nuances in the way their baby reacts to the stimuli they provide. By two or three months of age, the infant responds with surprise, for its nervous system is now geared to recognize unfamiliar gestures, voices, or toys. When three-month-old babies begin to smile at the human face, it is because at first they are not sure if it is a face they know, and then they assimilate it: "Oh, that's a human being; it looks like my mother. Ahh."

To be sure, the smile of assimilation is one of the earliest triggers of natural highs. Arielle's father describes how his parents reacted to their grandchild's first affirmations of their existence.

> Arielle is three months old. She enjoys feeding and being held, but she seems to show most pleasure when smiling at a loving human face. First a twinkle, . . . soon a smirk, . . . now a grin, cascading into a gurgling chortle of infant joy. Grandma giggles like a schoolgirl as Grandpa gleefully mimes one comical expression after another. A crescendo of shared laughter marks a new round of beckons and coos, until the next moment of exalted delight. Everyone is naturally high.

Around three months of age, the infant reaches out with its sensory system so that it can build a continuous picture of what the world is like. The smile of assimilation and the alert look of perplexity or surprise are possible only because the baby has already learned to distinguish between novel and familiar situations; if an infant sees the same thing over and over again, it becomes bored and will not look at it for very long. And by the age of six months, the baby has already formed definite categories and concepts regarding situations and people. Jerome Kagan of Harvard University describes this incredible need to take it all in, to assimilate and distinguish—the infant's quest for knowledge.

> It is very important to appreciate that the child is learning new information every day, because that is the way it is. . . . A well-fed seagull

on a summer afternoon will just fly around. It has no reason to fly around, but it does because that's the way seagulls are built. Human beings are built to seek new information, to learn from it, to consolidate that knowledge and move on.

Can a parent help to speed the infant's quest by, as Magnea puts it, "hearing all the little sounds, seeing all the little signals, and responding to them"? Certainly—especially if the parental response involves presenting the infant with more stimulating sights and sounds. In fact, all the available research indicates that children's early mental functioning is optimized by the presence of novel or stimulating toys or other objects. When children are exposed to variety and encouraged to explore their surroundings, intellectual functioning can flourish. Toys that seem most beneficial respond to infants' natural maneuvers—squeeze toys that squeak, bath toys that float, jack-in-the-boxes that jump.

There may well be a genetic component to the way an infant responds to this type of stimulation. Research, however, strongly suggests that when children are exposed to elements in their surroundings that are varied, interesting, and responsive—causing the child to stretch existing knowledge, yet not overly frustrating or challenging—intellectual functioning is further advanced.

Self-Discovery

Between one and a half and two years of age, healthy children become aware that they can have an effect on the world. The child begins to use the personal pronoun *I;* particularly among siblings, the possessive form appears, too. (No one has ever come up with a better way to assert ownership of a toy than the simple exclamation "Mine!") More important, children begin to realize that they have intentions, feelings, and actions; they are individuals, not just physically but mentally separated from others.

In a simple demonstration known as the rouge test, a three-month-old child whose nose has been dabbed with rouge looks in the mirror but will not touch the rouged nose, because the child does not connect the face in the mirror with his or her own face. By eighteen to twenty months, the child will touch the rouged nose, for the child has recently developed a sense of self—the result of his or her increasingly complex interactions with the rest of the world.

Another milestone in early development is the emergence of a moral sense. Well before the child's second birthday, the concept of "naughty" begins to appear. Children are bothered if they see something that is flawed or otherwise out of place. An eighteen-month-old child will say "broken," "dirty," or "mess"—particularly after tossing his or her bowl of cereal all over the floor. Here begins the lifelong process of comprehending that there is some order in the world, and when that order is violated, someone or something has done something wrong. The Terrible Twos are famous for the use of two powerful words—*self* and *no*—as in this exchange:

Father: Let Daddy tie your shoes.
Two-year-old: No. . . . Don't want to. . . . Self.

Once thought to be an obstreperous period of great obstinacy, psychologists now recognize the Terrible Twos as a time when the child begins to declare his or her independence and becomes engaged in the issue of establishing right from wrong.

During the next few years, children increasingly relate their concepts of how things work to abstract phenomena, like poverty in the outside world. At age four, Tasha discussed how coconuts could be a ready source of food for poor people who lived in the jungle: "They could climb a tree and bring back food for their families and friends." Seven-year-olds may develop theories for how to resolve problems of starvation, illness, or war.

As the child's concept of the world widens, elements of anxiety or fear begin to emerge. In Selma Fraiberg's landmark book *The Magic Years,* she describes how frightening fantasies are natural to a developing child. In a hypothetical example, a child named Frankie is designated by his parents to be the prototype of a modern, scientifically reared youngster. The probable sources of his fears are identified, and his parents devise schemes for their systematic decontamination: "Nursery rhymes and fairy tales were edited and revised; mice and their tails were never parted; and ogres dined on Cheerios instead of human flesh. . . . When Frankie's parakeet was stricken by a fatal disease, the corpse was removed and a successor installed before Frankie awakened from his afternoon nap." Despite all these precautions, Frankie persists in becoming afraid. At the age of two, he becomes concerned with going down the bathtub drain; unenthusiastic about the arrival of a new baby sister, he becomes pre-occupied with disposing of her at the local supermarket; and even though his parents have meticulously avoided violence, his dreams feature a series of giants, whom he conveniently eliminates by having their heads chopped off.

> It is not the bathtub drain, the dream about the giant, or the unpropitious arrival of a sibling that creates a neurosis. The future mental health of the child does not depend on the presence or absence of ogres in his fantasy life, or on such fine points as the diets of ogres. . . . *[I]t depends on the child's solution to the ogre problem.* It is the way in which the child manages his irrational fears that determines their effect on his personality development. . . . Normally, the child overcomes his irrational fears. And here is the most fascinating question of all . . . how does he do it?. . . Even in the second year he possesses a marvelously complex mental system which provides the means for anticipating danger, assessing danger, defending against danger and overcoming danger. Whether this equipment can be successfully employed by the child in overcoming his fears will depend, of course, on *the parents,* who in a sense, teach him to use his equipment.

To the extent that parents and other youth affiliates understand the nature of the developing child—especially those parts of his or her personality which strive toward conflict resolution and health—there is greater opportunity to assist in the formation of inner strengths and resources for dealing with life. The child's own sense of self will naturally undergo considerable revision and refinement before maturity; along the way, one of the greatest hurdles a child will face, a challenge in which the parents will inevitably play a significant role, has to do with the struggle to express and understand one's own emotions.

The Developing Child

Babies have feelings from the moment they are born. But their early emotional responses are limited to such basic expressions as surprise and distress. With the passage of time, however, an array of emotions begins to unfold in a series of predictable stages. Curiously, joy, which the infant can already display by six to eight weeks, has been found to precede sadness by many months.

It's not unusual for adults—even parents and teachers—to fall into the trap of judging children's emotional reactions by adult standards. Indeed, some adults seem to expect that children should display a full range of emotional sensitivity and restraint at an early age, a demand that effectively denies children the right to childlike behavior. Like everything else, the process of emotional maturation is a matter of degrees, and parents can reap considerable practical benefit from realizing just how gradual it is. Since humility, for example, is not usually part of the child's emotional repertoire until the age of five, the outlandish bragging of a four-year-old should be understood as quite natural ("Why, of *course* young Johnny can perform balancing acts, magic tricks, and extraordinary feats of strength—can't everybody?").

According to Terry Brazelton, a Harvard University researcher and popular author on child development, "It's about time we looked at emotions more carefully. Everything we know about a child shows that healthy emotional development is the key to other kinds of growth."

When the Feelings Arrive

Emotional capacities present at birth:

pleasure/surprise/disgust/distress

By 6–8 weeks:	joy
By 3–4 months:	anger
By 8–9 months:	sadness
	fear
By 12–18 months:	tender affection
By 18 months:	shame
By 2 years:	pride
By 3–4 years:	guilt
By 5–6 years:	social emotions, including insecurity, humility, confidence, and envy
By adolescence:	romantic passion
	philosophical brooding

The data represent average ages at which emotions are clearly present. Children vary.

Source: Joseph Campos at the University of Denver, and other researchers. Adapted from: *NY Times,* Science Times, June 19, 1984. Goleman, Daniel. "Order found in development of emotions." pp. 19–20.

From ages two to five, a child's life is marked by tremendous growth in all dimensions. When three-year-olds become less preoccupied with self-assertion ("Mine!"), they begin to push out energetically into the world, using all their sensory, imaginative, and creative faculties. At this age, the child initiates activities, always testing the rules of parents and society. When a child invents a game, it's a way of trying to see what the rules are, how we live by them, and how far one can go in one direction or another.

Around the age of four, children have already internalized their parents' voices and can be made to feel guilty about having impulses to explore limits and boundaries. Parental help and understanding permit self-direction to set sail, guided by a moral rudder that is neither too rigid nor too loose.

Studies of youngsters' artwork provide some indication of the leaps in mental development occurring at this age. By the time the young artist is four years old, his or her stick figures may acquire flesh and clothes, while the five-year-old, by contrast, can develop elaborate environments for his or her characters to explore and conquer. Physically, five-year-old children are more like adults: they display increased muscle tissue and a stronger and sturdier body, and perhaps most significant, their brain has reached 90 percent of its adult weight.

Play is the child's resource for dealing with his or her experiences and making sense out of the world. Like infants, preschool children are rooted in sensory impressions, but they can use ideas to explore how elements of their surroundings form logical and coherent systems. A four-year-old, for example, may pack a suitcase full of clothes and announce to her family that she is embarking on a train journey to "Pichoinki"—or some other exotic destination. On arrival, she continues, she plans to stay overnight at a hotel that has room only for her and her doll. Around the same time that they are piecing together such imaginative constructs, children are also likely to become intensely curious about (and comment on) physical differences between the sexes. In a preview of adult sexuality, they may develop an interest in having an exclusive—often possessive—relationship with the parent of the opposite sex.

During the elementary school years—ages six through twelve—children become preoccupied with personal accomplishments of all kinds. They enjoy doing and making many things, following projects to completion. It is not unusual to see a school-age child practice a sport or skill for many hours each day. One ten-year-old "Sultan of Swat," for example, would take his baseball gear out on the street and blast the ball from one end of the block to the other, for hours on end, perfecting his talent for hitting home runs.

During late childhood, the family remains important, but parents generally don't play as large a role in the child's life as they once did. Most children display a growing sense of independence, putting increasing energy into the pursuit of their own drives and social needs. Six hours per day are spent in school, much of the remaining time with friends or alone. While preschool children are egocentric, thinking only in terms of themselves, older children become concerned with the perceptions and feelings of others. When asked to describe a friend, a four-year-old may say, "He's naughty because he doesn't listen to my words," whereas an eight-year-old may begin to wonder how the other child regards him: "She likes me because I tell her funny stories." At school, children begin to develop academic and behavioral standards by which they compare themselves to their peers, and they strive for recognition in multiple spheres, tying their sense of self-worth to athletic, social, and academic achievement. Inevitably, this painful process causes even the most well-adjusted child to suffer periods of loneliness and self-doubt: "Is there something wrong with me?"

Social acceptance, or lack of it, also becomes an increasingly significant factor in the shaping of values and belief systems. The five-year-old's moral development tends to be guided by obedience to parental authority and the promise of future rewards. By age ten to twelve, however, a child's internal values are demonstrated through "good acts" and upholding social order. Children at this stage usually respond strongly to the threat of social stigma, with a distinct focus on peer approval. This socialization process is marked by an increased capacity to fathom abstract concepts; to the extent that children learn to relate "real-world" problems—such as war, pollution, poverty, and injustice—to their own lives, they start to take on new dimensions of personal and social responsibility.

Different cultures acknowledge this moral coming-of-age in various ways, but they all do. It is not simply a matter of coincidence that by seven years of age the Catholic church considers children old enough to confess, and English common law considers a child responsible for his crime. Parents in the Third World may entrust an entire herd of cattle to the watchful eye of a ten-year-old, while an eight-year-old may take care of her younger sister. (In Iceland, one of us became acquainted with a girl named Guri, who at age twelve was already a licensed babysitter.)

Unfortunately, the child's growing sense of social responsibility and involvement doesn't instantly lead to mature judgment or "right" behavior—far from it. Not only are adolescents powerfully influenced by peer behavior, but they are undergoing that exquisite and dramatic ritual of emotional and physical torture known as puberty. Most readers probably remember the basics (if not the agonizing embarrassment) from their health education classes. It takes the body an average of six years to complete sexual development. Girls begin to mature earlier than boys, with the onset of menstruation usually between the ages of twelve and thirteen. The pelvis widens to accommodate the birth process; protective layers of fat emerge; the breasts enlarge and develop. By seventeen, most females are sexually mature. Males also experience dramatic, disconcerting changes: at ages thirteen to fifteen, there is a jump in height and weight. Hormonal effects result in the emergence of body hair, voice changes, and increased muscle mass. By eighteen, most males are sexually mature.

Personality changes during this period of Sturm and Drang (German for "storm and stress") often correspond with sexual preoccupations. Particularly now, when sex drives and mating needs are in a vivid state of "stall," there is much self-evaluation and concern with appearance. Sixteen-year-olds may develop "imaginary audiences"—perceiving themselves as the center of everyone else's experience.

In the following, three teenagers describe how their moods are affected by fluctuating evaluations of how they look:

When I feel bad, I look in the mirror and think it's because I look bad. And then all day I think that everyone else thinks I look bad, too. But then when I feel good about myself—even though I might look hideous—if I think that I look decent, then I don't feel so much pressure.

I think that how you look at yourself is affected by what people tell you. In the morning, you can look in the mirror and think you look fine; then you go to school and someone will say, "Why are you wearing your hair like that?" Then you look at yourself again and you think, "God, I guess I didn't look OK."

What people say can affect your mood all day, especially if it's a guy you like. If you go to school and you think you look really cute that day, and the guy you like says something mean to you about the way you look, or doesn't say anything, doesn't notice you at all, doesn't talk to you, you are so bummed. . . . Ten million people can tell you that you look really cute, but if he says something mean, the whole day goes downhill.

Although emotions are characteristically topsy-turvy in adolescence, thinking becomes more complex, too. Young adults develop the capacity for hypothetical reasoning, deductions, and conclusions. They can ponder the future of the world and the history of the universe. Still, their concepts may be astonishingly simplistic. Adolescents are ripe to become true believers in black-or-white scientific, political, or religious ideologies. Even more paradoxical is the teenager's penchant for magical thought: "I can do things that others can't because I am special." This kind of logic is conducive to drug experimentation, skydiving, and teenage pregnancies. Conversely, some teenagers may overcome tremendous obstacles by parlaying idealism and zealous enthusiasm into enormous feats of artistry and strength. The dramatic movement between the heights of achievement and the depths of self-doubt can turn adolescence into a kind of roller-coaster ride of clashing emotions and beliefs. At fourteen, Romania's Nadia Comaneci stunned the world by winning three gold medals and scoring the first perfect 10s in Olympic gymnastics. At fifteen, she tried to kill herself by drinking bleach when the government forced her to leave her gymnastics coach.

The magical thinking characteristic of adolescence is of particular concern today because of the threat of AIDS. According to a survey of 3,000 high school seniors conducted by Who's Who among American High School Students in November 1992—three weeks after basketball superstar Magic Johnson revealed he had contracted the HIV virus—there was little change in the sexual practices of teenagers, despite their increased AIDS awareness. Although the proportion of teenagers who were "worried" or "very worried" about getting the HIV virus nearly doubled—from 12 to 22 percent—after Johnson's announcement, the number of students who said they "never" use condoms actually increased—from 8 to 12 percent. Among the 28 percent of surveyed students who indicated that they were sexually active, 42 percent said they would continue to have sexual intercourse even if a condom were not available.

The survey also revealed that many students did not openly discuss AIDS in their home or at school. Nearly one-fourth said they had not discussed the topic with teachers, and nearly one-third said there was no discussion of it in their families! Yet virtually every health professional who has studied the problem agrees that the key to controlling the spread of AIDS depends on providing our children with solid information on how the disease is contracted and the appropriate precautions to take to minimize one's risk of becoming infected. Parents can't afford to engage in their own "magical thinking" by ignoring their children's seeming ignorance of or indifference to AIDS and other serious health threats. The responsibilities of nurturing healthy children extend into adolescence—for example, in initiating direct and sensitive discussion of AIDS well before children become sexually active. Until a cure or vaccine is found, our strongest ally is education.

There are four known ways of contracting AIDS: through unprotected sex, through blood transfusions, from mother to child during fetal development, and through sharing hypodermic needles. While blood transfusions are no longer a significant risk in the United States, and approximately two-thirds of babies who are born HIV positive no longer test positive several months after birth, intravenous drug users and unprotected sexual partners remain highly vulnerable. Parents should consider urging their children to delay sex until marriage, or at least until they have made a "serious commitment," but should also be realistic about the likelihood that their children will at some point engage in casual sex. Children who may experiment with sex can benefit from information about how to procure condoms, as well as instructions regarding their proper use—and their limitations. (While we're on the topic, another vital area of discussion with young people involves addressing their unfounded concerns regarding AIDS transmission. People do not get AIDS from holding hands with, going to school with, playing ball with, or casually befriending carriers of the HIV virus or people with AIDS.)

Only by providing direct, no-nonsense information about everything from the importance of condoms to the need for compassion and sensitivity toward AIDS sufferers can we hope to combat the disastrous effects of magical thinking. AIDS is very much the tragedy of the moment, but the fact is that young people's tendency to view themselves as invincible ("It'll never happen to me!"), their fondness for magical thinking, is a timeless folly. In Aristotle's words,

> The young are in character prone to desire and ready to carry any desire they may have formed into action. Of bodily desire it is the sexual to which they are most disposed to give way, and in regard to sexual desire they exercise no self-restraint. They are changeful, too, and fickle in their desires, which are as transitory as they are vehement; for their wishes are keen without being permanent, like a sick man's fits of hunger and thirst.
>
> They are passionate, irascible, and apt to be carried away by their impulse. They are the slave too of their passion, as their ambition prevents their ever brooking a slight and renders them indignant at the mere idea of enduring an injury.... They are fonder both of honor and victory than of money, the reason why they care so little for money being that they have never yet had experience of want.
>
> They are charitable rather than the reverse, as they have never yet been witness of many villainies; and they are trustful as they have not yet been often deceived.... They have high aspirations; for they have never yet been humiliated by the experience of life, but are unacquainted with the limiting force of circumstances....
>
> If the young commit a fault, it is always on the side of excess and exaggeration, for they carry everything too far, whether it be their love or hatred or anything else. They regard themselves as omniscient and are positive in their assertions; this is in fact, the reason of their carrying everything too far.

Nurturing healthy children by guiding them through critical phases of development has benefits throughout life—yours and theirs. Indeed, natural highs—positive feeling states triggered by the integration of thoughts, activities, and personal values—depend on the positive resolution of specific psychological conflicts, and that can come only through such nurturing. Otherwise, energy is directed to problems that were not effectively handled during childhood. An adult, for example, who failed to establish trust in his parents, resulting in an enduring lack of confidence in his associates, may find great difficulty in finding happiness in his work or his home life.

Erik and Joan Erikson, now in their tenth decade, postulate that lessons from each of life's stages mature into multiple facets of wisdom that blossom during old age. As shown in Table 2.1, positive attributes (e.g., hope, will, purpose) that are generated from the res-

TABLE 2.1

The Completed Life Cycle of Natural Highs

Conflict and Resolution	Attribute	Attainment in Old Age
Old age Integrity vs. despair	Wisdom	Existential identity; a sense of identity strong enough to withstand physical disintegration
Adulthood Generativity vs. stagnation	Care	*Caritas,* caring for others; and *agape,* empathy and concern
Early adulthood Intimacy vs. isolation	Love	Sense of the complexity of relationships; value of tenderness and loving freely
Adolescence Identity vs. confusion	Fidelity	Sense of complexity of life; merger of sensory, logical, and aesthetic perceptions
School age Industry vs. inferiority	Competence	Humility; acceptance of the course of one's life and unfulfilled hopes
Play age Initiative vs. guilt	Purpose	Humor; empathy; resilience
Early childhood Autonomy vs. shame	Will	Acceptance of the cycle of life, from integration to disintegration
Infancy Basic trust vs. mistrust	Hope	Appreciation of interdependence and relatedness

Source: Adapted from: *NY Times,* Science Times, June 14, 1988. Goleman, Daniel. "Erikson in his old age expands his view of life." pp. 13–14.

olution of specific psychological conflicts culminate in a strong sense of purpose and meaning, even in the face of death.

Unhealthy Families

The complex interplay of biological, psychological, and cultural transformations makes youth a particularly vulnerable time of life. We can, however, learn a great deal about the emerging personality by looking not simply at the effects of these influences on the individual, but at the soundness of the surrounding family structure, the "good home" in which these dramatic changes occur. If personality represents the combined influence of genetic and environmental factors, then to a great extent the family is responsible for both.

Family systems theory views human functioning in terms of relationships, rather than focusing on the individual. The family is seen as a living system—an emotional organism—with each individual as a component part. If there is change in one part of the structure (i.e., change in a family member's role), it must be compensated for elsewhere in the system. In alcoholic families, for example, when the drinking member becomes sober, others in the family may begin to experience distress.

Unhealthy families are often governed in an authoritarian manner by one strong leader, who imposes order and conformity at the expense of individuals. There may be blatant disrespect for the uniqueness of family members. For example, Homer Simpson, the boorish dad in the popular animated television series "The Simpsons," gives his wife, Marge, a bowling ball for her thirty-fourth birthday—with *his* name on it. Although he learns to regret it, the self-centered gesture is characteristic of the kind of distorted values and conduct portrayed by the show, which has displayed an alarmingly on-target ability to mirror and satirize the worst aspects of unhealthy family interaction in America.

In the world of "The Simpsons," as in far too many real-life families, rules are made for someone else's benefit (usually the rule maker's) and not for the good of the person who must keep them. Spontaneity and creativity are discouraged, because authoritarian parents make little allowance for separate personalities or extenuating circumstances. Sanctions are often unrealistic and/or impossible to keep; they encourage dishonesty—with self and others—in an effort to avoid punishment or rejection. When Bart Simpson gets beaten by a bully, his father, Homer, advises, "Never say anything unless you're sure everyone feels exactly the same way." Communication problems are rampant: secrets are kept; emotions are hidden, invalidated, or denied. Marge Simpson passes on the secret of popularity to her daughter, Maggie, when she tells her, "Just smile. Then you'll fit in and you'll be invited to parties and the boys will like you and happiness will follow."

One of the fundamental obstacles to healthy relationships is a phenomenon that psychologists call "lack of boundaries"—generally, family situations in which the individual members fail to properly acknowledge individual needs and limits. Unhealthy families tend to become either "walled" or "enmeshed." In walled families, interpersonal barriers are so thick that there can be no true interaction or intimacy between family members. A father refuses to sanction his son's anger or grief over the death of a pet, for example, and simply urges him to "be a man"; a mother is intensely uncomfortable with her daughter's emerging sexuality or her spouse's alcoholism but out of shame or fear refuses to confront the issue. Such families are characterized by high anxiety, loneliness, rigidity, and lack of mutual respect.

When families are too tightly knit, wholesome interpersonal distances are nearly impossible to maintain. Enmeshed families enact chronic violations of personal boundaries, physical and otherwise. There's no separation between "good" touching (a fatherly hug) and "bad" touching (molestation or child abuse), or between one's own beliefs and feelings and those of other family members. Since each family member is an extension of the others, there are no whole people to relate to; therefore, true intimacy is impossible. Chronic anxiety is also a hallmark of these families, a consequence of overlapping roles and confused, covert rules.

Even in the most supportive families, separation is a difficult process. Parents can be so generous that they serve only in limiting their child's experience. Sheltered childhoods deny young people the opportunity to master basic life skills, such as procuring a job or managing a household. Alan and Beth Sims, for example, have three children, ages twenty to twenty-six, all living at home. Janet, twenty, the youngest, attends college and has never had to work, except for making her bed to claim a hearty allowance. Her monthly expenditures for clothing and school costs exceed $2,000. Todd, twenty-three, also attends college, and has been promised a jeep if he can manage a 3.5 grade point average. But the most problematic child is Paul, twenty-six, who started a disc jockey business from the home. He pays no rent and receives calls throughout the night inquiring about his company, "Burst of Light." Today, 59 percent of men and 47 percent of women between eighteen and twenty-four years of age depend on their parents for housing. Legions of frustrated parents are torn between the natural urge to launch their children into autonomous living and weighty concerns regarding their physical and emotional well-being.

> And a woman who held a babe against her bosom said, "Speak to us of Children."
>
> And he said, "Your children are not your children. They are the sons and daughters of Life's longing for itself. They come through you but not from you, and though they are with you, yet they belong not to you. You may give them your love but not your thoughts. You may house their bodies but not their souls, for their souls dwell in the house of tomorrow, which you cannot visit, not even in your dreams. You may strive to be like them, but seek not to make them like you. For life goes not backward nor tarries with yesterday. You are the bows from which your children as living arrows are sent forth. The archer sees the mark upon the path of the infinite, and He bends you with His might that His arrows may go swift and far. Let your bending in the archer's hand be for gladness; for even as He loves the arrow that flies, so He loves also the bow that is stable."
>
> —Kahlil Gibran

How do we strike a balance between appropriate support and the kind of emotional smothering that, however well intentioned, can deflect the arrow from its path? Some find humor an extraordinary means for gaining perspective, as well as for opening delicate conversations with or about young people. Consider the following as one example of how "lightening up" can get a family closer to direct communication about the troublesome issues that arise during early adulthood:

Letter from a College-Age Daughter to Her Parents

Dear Mom and Dad,

My first month in college has been very exciting, and I'm very sorry for not having written sooner. I'm going to tell you everything that's happened, but could you please have a seat before we go on. OK?

Right now, I'm doing fairly well. The head injury that I got when I jumped off the dorm roof, which was engulfed in flames last Saturday night, is almost all better. I was in the hospital for ten days, and now I don't get dizzy anymore.

Luckily, the dorm is located near our sewage treatment facility, and one of the workers saw me jump. As a matter of fact, he was the one who first saw the fire, then called the ambulance, and rode with me all the way to the hospital.

And guess what! Since the dorm was completely demolished and I was basically out on the street, he had the generosity to share his apartment with me. Actually, it's an attic in a nearby tenement building, but he did a great job decorating. He's a real sweetie, and I love him with all my heart. We're engaged to get married, although I'm not sure about the exact date, but it has to be soon because the pregnancy will probably show in the next few months.

That's right, Mom and Dad, I'm pregnant! Isn't it great? You've always wanted to be grandparents, and I know how thrilled you'll be to help me look after the baby, just like you took care of me when I was a child.

The reason that we haven't been able to set the marriage date is that my boyfriend has a minor infection, which, although it's really no big deal, will prevent us from passing the premarital blood tests. And so I caught it from him.

I know you'll invite him into our family with all the love and kindness you have given to your own children. He is very gentle, and even though he doesn't have a high school diploma, he really works very hard. I'm sure that his race and religious beliefs, which are different from ours, won't bother you at all, since you've always been so open-minded.

Now that I've explained everything to you, I want to confess that the dormitory fire never really happened. I didn't have any head injury or dizziness. I am neither engaged nor pregnant. I don't have a new boyfriend, and I'm not infected; but I am getting a D in biology and flunking English literature. I just want you to see these grades in their proper perspective.

Healthy Families

It's far easier, of course, to describe the attributes of faulty parents than to establish guidelines for nurture and support. Effective parenting—the foundation of healthy families—is a formidable challenge. Jerome Kagan tells us:

> I think the basic ingredients really are tremendous respect for the integrity of each child, a belief that each child has very special qualities and that those qualities will be expressed under appropriate kinds of

conditions. And that teaching doesn't mean directing or imposing; it really means opening up or liberating.

. . . There is no formula. There is no easy way to do this. There is no single way to do it. The gift of teaching and the gift of parenting is one that has to be rediscovered with each child.

Julio and Ada Rodriguez are immigrants from Lima, Peru. Together they have eight children, three boys and five girls, who range from seventeen to thirty-two years of age. In 1989, because of political turmoil and a growing sense of danger, they established residence with the four youngest girls in West Palm Beach, Florida. The family is remarkable, in that each member exudes warmth and self-confidence while enjoying exceptional balance in work, love, and play.

The eldest boy, Julio Eduardo, is a graduate student at the Colorado School of Mines; Marissa, age thirty-, lives with her husband and two children, ages five and three, in Lima; Cecilia, twenty-six, has a master's degree in business administration; Carlos, twenty-four, who attended medical school in Mexico, is married to a Mexican native, has a five-year-old daughter, and plans to complete a residency in surgery in the United States; Julio Cesar, twenty-two, is happily married and living in Chicago; Jessica, twenty, is attending the University of Michigan, studying psychology and political science; Monica, eighteen, attends Palm Beach Community College and is interested in pediatric medicine; and Lilliana, seventeen, a high school senior, wants to be a physician with a specialty in obstetrics.

How did this family get off to such a good start? How did they manage to transcend the upheaval of leaving their homeland while continuing to lead creative, responsible, and family-centered lives? Julio, who at the age of fifty-six already has three grandchildren, attributes success to family cohesion, spiritual guidance, and respect for physical health. None of the children smokes cigarettes, and the few who drink any alcohol at all do so in moderation.

We were a very close family and had very conservative ideas. The children were taught to be Catholic and that they should take care of their bodies and minds in order to achieve happiness. We always stressed involvement in some kind of exercise—athletics, running, or jogging as a family—while trying to give them pride in being a

Rodriguez. Also, we understood that we would always be joined to-gether. I told them we should be like a tree. We like each other and are always in touch and know what is happening in the family. When there is an important matter, we all talk about it together.

We like them to be involved with games like chess, to make their minds sharp. I encouraged them to read anything, especially the clas-sics: *Little Women* for the girls; for the boys, a book called *Corazon,* or *Heart,* about Italian boys who came with their family to Argentina. It shows how the family gets together. My library has at least 120 classics. We read *Don Quixote, Ivanhoe* and other world literature, while exposing them to scientific information as well. Also, I encour-age them to listen to good music and appreciate fine paintings. We try to go at least once a year to the theater or opera.

Ada Rodriguez interrupted her career to stay home with the chil-dren.

Yes. . . . Before, I was an elementary school teacher. Then when I had the children, I stayed home. What makes me most happy is to be to-gether with the family, to help them grow and to give them anything they need. When they were children, we tried to work together as a team, to help them resolve their problems. The role of the mother is the most important in the family, because the children need to be cared for all the time. Little by little, they learn what Mother wants for them, and they need a lot of help; they need many kinds of things. Sometimes I wonder why I didn't continue teaching. But I feel it was best that I stopped then. Now I may go back to teaching, to work for myself, now that they are grown.

Cecilia, twenty-eight, the oldest child still living at home, de-scribes how she takes pleasure in simple but vital activities that cul-tivate relationships and a deep personal sense of well-being—her own version of natural highs.

One of the ways I do it is just talking to people, writing letters—I love to write—exercises, studying, walking. I'm not very sociable in terms of making friends, but I have a few deep, lasting relationships. It was nice to be on my own, but now, being back with the family, I recog-nize that you need the other part. . . . There is someone always there that you can count on, that you can talk to, or just do things together.

Monica, eighteen, the next-to-youngest child, finds that Ameri-cans like to smoke and drink. She prefers going to parties without alcohol or drugs, enjoying the exhilaration of dancing to reggae and salsa music with her Spanish-speaking friends. Lilliana and Jessica find singing a rewarding form of creativity and self-expression. Cecilia has her own theories about how the kids were able to avoid the common adolescent bouts with substance abuse.

> Maybe what helped was the fact that it wasn't any trouble to drink in my house. When we were little, we used to have a glass of wine; it wasn't forbidden. So I tried, just like any other kid, and there was a time maybe that I got drunk. And I realized it wasn't fun. Also, I was one of the two children who smoked in my family. I probably did it because the people around me smoked and it was cool. But it wasn't difficult for me to quit, because I knew that it wasn't something I really needed to do.

Obviously, this account of the Rodriguez family is not intended as a cookbook for how to create an optimal family. Many women, for example, would be neither comfortable remaining at home nor financially able to do so, ministering to the needs of eight youngsters. Still, putting aside the specifics of religion and cultural preferences, there are some general principles concerning the healthy family that the Rodriguezes exemplify.

Burton White and Michael Meyerhoff, of the Center for Parent Education in Newton, Massachusetts, have spent nearly two decades researching the qualities of good parents. Most important, they found, was the thoroughly unsurprising revelation that healthy parents are able to give their children a deep feeling of love. This involves providing warm, secure contact during the first years of life, but also paramount is the ability to provide fair yet firm and consistent discipline when required. Self-esteem is preserved through honest and open communication. Effective parents are able to set clear limits, without abandoning their high standards for fear of losing a child's affection or loyalty. Appropriate praise is vital.

Independent of possessing elaborate toys, or of adhering to a well-organized educational plan, well-adjusted children have parents who appreciate how exciting and novel nearly everything is, who receive with enthusiasm and encouragement every new achievement of the developing child—from simple movements, like clapping hands, to early signs of creative self-expression, as in fingerpainting, to the lightninglike growth of ideas and expression that follows. By the same token, children who are encouraged to become involved in activities and events that routinely exist throughout the household can find, as William Blake so aptly put it, "the world in a grain of sand . . . and eternity in an hour." Challenge, stimulation, and creativity exist side by side with limits, consistency, and predictability.

According to Virginia Satir, families and their constituent members thrive when provided with what she terms the "Five Freedoms":

    I. The freedom to see and hear what is here and now, rather than what was, what will be or should be.

   II. The freedom to think and know what one thinks and knows, rather than what one should think and know.

  III. The freedom to feel and express what one feels, rather than what one should feel and express.

  IV. The freedom to want and to choose what one wants, rather than what one should want.

   V. The freedom to imagine one's own self-actualization, rather than playing a rigid role or always playing it safe.

Of special note is that good parents act as personal consultants to their kids, rather than doubling as surrogate teachers. They promote and enrich activities with which their children become occupied. Instead of controlling or taking over, they elaborate or give simple help when requested. A father describes how he acted as consultant to his four-year-old daughter when she first learned to swim:

> I knew it was important when Tasha declined to watch a kid's video after dinner.
>
> "No!" said Tasha. "I want to show Daddy how I can swim without using a float or water wings."
>
> As soon as we got to the pool, she ran off a whole agenda of swimming feats.
>
> "What should I do?" I said.
>
> "You don't have to do anything. Just watch. Now go over there."
>
> So, following her lead, I entered the pool and maneuvered to about six feet away. Without hesitating, she lowered herself in the pool and began paddling toward me, her body at about a forty-five degree angle to the surface, mouth just barely above the water. Except for her tiny chin, Tasha's adorable little head was bobbing above water.
>
> I had to refrain from making an uncalled-for parental rescue. So I stayed put. The few seconds of waiting became flooded with excite-

ment. When she lunged into my arms, her tiny body was ecstatic—hugs and kisses.

"See, Daddy, I can swim."

The next half-hour was filled with a series of practice lessons designed by my ebullient tadpole. First swimming without any props, then using a tiny float, then going underwater for a two-second dive, then swimming again without any float, then using the regular float—all the time measuring distances and progress. When I mentioned that we must be getting cold, because our lips were chattering, her knowing reply was, "Gotta keep moving, Daddy!"

Health Promotion at School

Educational philosophy has become an increasingly relevant issue in nurturing healthy children, particularly as our schools have taken on a more significant role in child development. Not only are children enrolled in programs at younger ages—many from infancy—but the length of the program day for all ages has been extended to accommodate the needs of employed families. This expansion of the school's role has been marked by a growing emphasis on formal instruction. At the same time, we're hearing from contemporary researchers that children learn most effectively through play.

The National Association for the Education of Young Children (NAEYC), which represents the consensus of early childhood professionals, believes that "a high-quality early childhood program promotes the physical, social, emotional and cognitive development of young children while responding to the needs of families." To the extent that there are universal, predictable sequences of growth and change that occur in children during the first decade of life, teachers may create complementary learning environments and plan age-appropriate experiences. Ideally, such planning should also be responsive to individual differences; it should have sufficient flexibility to take into account the uniqueness of each child, individual growth patterns, special interest areas, and cultural leanings, so that teachers can design the most beneficial learning environment. And play—the forerunner of future natural highs—is the staple of positive early education programs.

How do we go about laying the in-school groundwork for natural highs? Of primary importance during kindergarten and the early grades is child-initiated, child-directed, teacher-supported play. Curricula at early levels should be able to accommodate a chronological age range of as much as two years for any group. Such broad scope requires a rich diversity of teaching materials, methods, and room assignments. Basic learning materials include sand, water, clay, and accessories to use with them. (Although frequent use of pictures and stories helps build on children's real experiences, workbooks and coloring books are not appropriate for children under six years of age—they may stifle the child's spontaneous learning responses.) The learning environment may also include blocks; puzzles; games; manipulative toys; dramatic play props, such as those for housekeeping and transportation; science investigation equipment; books and recordings; and water-based paint and other devices for creative expression.

Amid this hearty array of learning tools, teachers facilitate child development by increasing the challenge of activity through timely questions and suggestions, or by adding more complex materials and ideas as children become involved. In order to integrate physical and intellectual growth with the child's emotional needs, teachers may develop a set of classroom responsibilities, such as helping with food service or cleanup routines, always supporting positive interactions and problem-solving opportunities with other children and adults.

From day care until well into adolescence, educational activities should be guided by what we know about how children *learn* as much as by any other criteria. Infants and toddlers learn by experiencing the environment through their senses, through physical movement and social interaction; hiding things and playing naming games are important at this stage. Talking and singing and presenting children with interesting sights and sounds open the channels of assimilation, too. As infants become more mobile, they use toys, language, and other learning materials. Warm, positive relationships with adults help them develop trust and a sense of self-esteem. Preschool marks the beginning of independence skills, including feeding, dressing, and going to the toilet. During the early stages of language development, preschoolers benefit from self-initiated repetition, as when the child of not quite two bids goodbye to her mother: "See ya soo . . . oon, Mo . . . mmy; see ya soo . . . oon."

From ages two through eight, the development of language, increased concentration and reasoning skills, and a burgeoning capacity to interact with physical and social environments become major factors in the educational process:

- Two-year-olds need simple books, pictures, puzzles, music, and room for active play. Groups of toddlers require more than one of each toy, since they do not yet comprehend sharing; even with multiples of the same toy, they can argue about who gets the right color.
- As three-year-olds grow more sturdy, large-muscle activities can be encouraged through such devices as climbers, blocks, and wheel toys. At this stage, they are able to benefit from listening to simple stories and taking part in basic conversations.
- Four-year-olds can perform small-motor activities, such as those involving scissors, art, and cooking. They concentrate better and can recognize the color or size of objects. Elementary math concepts and problem-solving skills may begin to develop. A four-year-old, for example, may become the self-initiated gatekeeper for a bundle of M&Ms and divide the booty among his or her friends by repeatedly counting out five pieces for each member of the group.
- Five-year-olds, who by now are beginning to recognize meaningful words and have often mastered writing their names, get more out of a print-rich environment than from simply learning the alphabet. Their increased attention span and shifting focus to events in the outside world allow for the planning of special events and field trips.
- Six-year-olds, who by now are developing problem-solving skills from playing games that involve increasingly complex rules, do well with hands-on activities, such as following directions to complete an artistic project.
- From age seven to eight, social interest becomes piqued, complemented by the child's increased skills at logic and reasoning. At this time, reading books that relate to the child's own experiences becomes a powerful method of learning. Similarly, math concepts may be understood through real-life calculations, as in cooking or carpentry.

Most educators would agree that, at each stage, adult-child interactions should be appropriate not only to each child's age but to his or her cultural background. It is important to provide multicultural and nonsexist experiences. Adults need to provide a balance of rest and activity throughout the program day, too, with the youngest receiving morning and/or afternoon naps; even older children need alternating periods of quiet and activity. Children should never be rushed, and schedules should be flexible enough to take advantage of impromptu experiences. Appropriate guidance of young children is based on respect. It helps to expect common types of behavior, such as messiness, interest in body parts and genital differences, crying and resistance, aggression—and, later, infraction of rules and truth.

Age-appropriate communication is important, too. During nursery school and preschool, adults should respond immediately to infants' cries of distress. The response should be warm and soothing as the adult identifies the child's needs. Grown-ups should also respond to infants' vocalizations, as well as to their manipulating of objects and movement, as these are the ways infants communicate. Holding, touching, making frequent eye contact, talking, and singing in a soothing tone are all helpful ways to relate to infants. Toddlers and two-year-olds need to have adults close at hand for attention and physical comfort. Adults can help assure them that they are understood by repeating or rephrasing words; the older the child, the more verbal responses can be. Positive cues like smiles and concentrated attention are important, with the adult sitting low or kneeling, making frequent eye contact, or moving quietly in a friendly and relaxed manner. Children develop communication skills by actively hearing and talking, not by being talked at. Individual and small-group interactions work best with preschoolers, where there can be one-on-one or at least two-way communication.

With regard to discipline, one should always bear in mind Carl Menninger's sage advice: "What's done to children, they will do to society." Teachers should promote frequent contact with families, sharing information about each child's progress or problem behavior. Through parent-teacher collaboration, mutual understanding and greater consistency can be achieved. Above all, mistakes should be valued as learning opportunities. Effective limit-setting includes redirecting children's unwanted behavior, listening respectfully to expressions of feelings and frustrations, modeling problem-solving skills, and explaining rules when necessary. Some adult behaviors are never acceptable in a school setting: screaming in anger; neglecting a child; inflicting physical or emotional pain; criticizing a child's person or family by ridiculing, blaming, teasing, insulting, or engaging in name-calling; threatening; and using frightening or humiliating punishment. Adults should neither laugh at children nor discuss their behavior in the presence of other kids. And last but not least, labeling or categorizing should be carefully avoided. Although it is sometimes necessary to identify intellectual, emotional, or behavioral traits for planning purposes, children tend to become what they are called. A frustrated dancer, for example, often referred to her six-year-old as clumsy, and she produced just that—a child who lacked self-confidence and was physically awkward and socially immature.

Adolescents are particularly sensitive to the criticisms they receive at home and in school. When teenagers were asked to describe the qualities of teachers that make them feel good or bad, they offered the following:

> We have this one English teacher and he's always calling us "retards" and stuff. He'll say, "Well, I've never taught an advanced class that has this many stupid people in it!" He's always telling us how stupid we are and that we could do things better. And sometimes we can do things better; sometimes we don't try as hard as we could. But still, when he comes in and says, "How are my retards?" I just want to hit him. He's always picking on people in class.
>
> Once we were having this discussion in class and everyone was giving their opinion on something and reasons for their opinions. Tim gave his, and it wasn't the most brilliant answer he could have given; and that teacher said, "Well, that's just a bunch of bullshit. Your opinion doesn't matter." And nobody said anything. With this teacher, we're all afraid he'll say something worse back. I don't even raise my hand in his class. I just try not to get called on, because I don't want him to sit there and talk about how stupid I am. You know, you think you're doing your best and you say your answer, and he'll say, "That's stupid." Then he doesn't say anything else; he just calls on somebody else, and you just sit there feeling stupid.
>
> But there are teachers who will encourage you and let you participate. They'll talk to you on a one-to-one basis, and you feel really comfortable talking to them. You can talk to them on the same level you talk to a friend. That's what really brings you up—when you go into one of those classes, you can be really open, say what's on your mind, let them know you're having a stressful day. Those teachers care about your whole life—not just your school life. They know your

outside life affects you. If they know you're doing sports, they'll say, "How did you do in your game?" That really helps. You can tell they're not just there to make you do the work. They are there for you if you have problems.

Even though teachers are important to the development of self-esteem, the greatest responsibility in the seemingly never-ending job of promoting a positive self-image is in the hands of the parents. And by listening to these kids, we discover that, for the most part, parents haven't changed much over the last generation or two. They are still comparing children to one another, siblings, cousins, and even themselves as teenagers; and these kids hate it as much as or even more than we did when we were their age.

> Well, with me, I feel I have to live up to my sister because I'm in the same classes that she was in when she was a sophomore, and I think I'm doing better than she did then. But since she's in college now and has a 4.0, my dad keeps saying, "Well, your sister has a 4.0 in college. Why can't you get a 4.0 in high school?" My mom compares me to the way she was when she was younger. She always talks about what a good student she was, how thin she was, and says, "I used to be thick like you and then I lost all my weight" and "I never tried to be dishonest with my mothers and I never did this, and I never did that." But I'm not her. I'm different. Also, she always wanted to play the piano when she was little, and her family didn't have the money so she could take lessons. So now she's making me do it. But I don't want to; I can't stand playing the piano.

Most of all, children want to be treated fairly. By the time they've reached their teens, they have reasonably sophisticated notions of social and family justice. Here's a familiar lament, a teenage girl expressing her frustration concerning her treatment by her parents relative to her three younger brothers:

> I was not allowed to go to the school dance—my eighth-grade dance. I went out and bought a dress and got a perm and all this stuff, and I was so excited to go. Then my parents didn't even let me go, because they made me go to our church—to this festival—and make shish kebabs. So I was at my church making shish kebabs while everyone else was at the dance. That really brought me down.
> But my brothers were always allowed to go out to dances. They

could go out to parties, to movies. They could do anything, because they're guys. My mom would say, "No, you're a girl and you have to act like a girl and girls don't go out. You're going to have a bad reputation." That's the only thing my mom cares about—my reputation.

I was talking to my mom about it the other day, and I told her, "I still hate you for what you did to me in the eighth grade." And she said, "Oh yeah, I understand. You're going to be scarred for life. But what can I do about it now?" They don't even understand now what they did to me.

When teenagers were asked how their parents might help them to feel good about themselves, they offered the following:

Talk to us, really talk to us. Every day. Ask us what we're doing, what we like to do; tell us when we're doing something wrong, but try to do it in a positive way; use constructive criticism, but be honest. Give us a lot of praise, but don't overdo it—you can take that too far and a kid can think that everything they do is perfect and better than everybody else.

Establishing Healthy Environments

Most of us think of health education as a field that focuses on reducing the risk of illness through narrowly defined physical efforts, such as maintaining a high-fiber, low-fat diet; engaging in regular aerobic exercise; using safety belts; refraining from smoking; and avoiding excessive alcohol consumption. Society appears to be stuck in an overly concrete physiological view of wellness. We seem to be trapped in the naive idea that by eating whole-grain cereals and getting aerobic, health and well-being will be at our doorstep. But important as maintaining physical health may be, it represents only the bottom tier of a comprehensive health promotion strategy. According to the widely quoted definition devised by the World Health Organization, health is "a state of complete physical, mental and social well being and not merely the absence of disease or infirmity."

A more sophisticated approach to "complete mental and social well being" would widen the focus of health education to include the state of our surrounding environment. This includes the physical environment in which we live (geography, architecture, and technology), the social ambience (determined by culture, economics, and politics), and such personal qualities as genetic predispositions and individual coping styles. All of these influences have a profound effect on the well-being not only of individual members of the community but of society itself. A program that aims to promote human health demands appreciation of the interplay between all these factors, with an eye toward what could be called "environmental intervention."

One form of environmental intervention that is gaining increasing media attention is the trend toward community-oriented policing, a concept developed by Herman Goldstein of the University of Wisconsin Law School. Conventional police strategy is "incident-oriented"—a victim or observer calls in an incident, such as a robbery or burglary, and the police respond by trying to apprehend the perpetrator. In a community-oriented approach, in addition to trying to catch the offender, police attempt to remedy the existing ecological conditions that contribute to criminal activity.

When the New Briarfield Apartments, a slum area in Newport News, Virginia, reported a rash of burglaries in 1984, Detective Tony Duke decided to interview the neighborhood residents about their problems. He found that, in addition to their obvious concern about crime, they were equally upset about the physical deterioration of their living quarters. Barry Haddix, the patrol officer assigned to the area, began working with a network of city agencies to fix up the project pending its eventual replacement. Garbage was systematically hauled away, potholes were filled, broken windows were replaced, and the streets were swept clean. Graffiti were painted over or wiped clean. A study conducted by the Police Executive Research Forum (PERF) indicates that the burglary rate at the New Briarfield Apartments dropped by 35 percent after the neighborhood improvement work was initiated.

This kind of police effort—coordinating social service and public health intervention agencies to alleviate some of the ecological conditions associated with crime—is going on in cities throughout America. According to neighborhood crime reporters James Q. Wilson and George L. Kelling, "This pattern constitutes the beginnings of the most significant redefining of police work in the past half century." Wilson and Kelling explain the apparent success of community-oriented police work by using a simple analogy concerning broken windows. If the first broken window is not repaired, then the people who enjoy destroying property will assume that nobody cares, and more windows will be broken until there are no more windows. Similarly, disorderly behavior—for example, crude or harassing remarks by alienated youngsters—will, if left unchallenged, signify lack of concern; the misbehavior may soon escalate to serious crime.

Of course, stimulating the interagency cooperation necessary to solve the initial "broken window" episode is itself a formidable challenge. In his book *Neighborhood Services,* John Mudd calls this the "Rat Problem":

> If a rat is found in an apartment, it is a housing inspection responsibility; if it runs into a restaurant, the Health Department has jurisdiction; if it goes outside and dies in the alley, Public Works takes over.

A police officer who becomes seriously involved in the public's concern about rats will go mad trying to discern what municipal agency has responsibility for rat control and then inducing it to kill rats. Nonetheless, police are persevering on an optimistic note. Community-oriented policing means reorganizing the law enforcement routine to include exploring and resolving emergent problems as well as reacting to illegal incidents. It means that whatever public consensus considers a threat to community order is therefore a "problem." It means working with, supporting, and promoting the good guys and not just chasing down or eliminating the bad guys.

But the idea of environmental intervention isn't limited to simply improving our own neighborhoods; living in a relatively stable community doesn't entirely insulate one from problems across town or across the world. Today we live in a global village spanned by vast electronic information networks—a situation that tends to both expand and distort our perceptions of what constitutes culture and social values. "The Day We Speak Peace" project exemplifies how concerns regarding our social ambience can be expressed on a global level. Originated by Marianne Weidlein of Boulder, Colorado, the project aims to organize a million people worldwide, all trying to influence the media to focus one day on life-affirming rather than violent news.

> Most of our news is about the atrocities, difficulties, problems, and tragedies that happen . . . about what is wrong, who to blame and

why, and even how they will be punished. Television programming and entertainment is more often of discord and violence than creative, inspiring stories and messages. Even our children's cartoons are permeated with violence and retribution. . . .

Is there a relationship between the quality of our news, programming, and entertainment, and the increased crime we are experiencing? . . .

Think how different life would be if our news and programming were more inspiring, creative and fun.

The major objection to television from parents and educators centers on the heavy dosage of media-portrayed sex and violence. It may seem unlikely that watching cartoon characters flatten one another could cause children to behave aggressively, but a large body of research on the relationship between television viewing and aggression indicates that this does, in fact, occur.

In a 1982 report published in the *American Psychologist,* L. D. Eron described how and when TV violence begins to influence children. He found that around the age of eight, children become more susceptible to what they see on the screen. The degree to which they are affected depends on how closely they identify with the program's characters and how realistic they believe the programs to be. Those children who watch violent TV are consistently rated as more aggressive by their peers.

Television networks often try to refute this kind of evidence by arguing that TV violence has a socially redeeming quality because the child learns the principle of good winning over evil. Not so, according to Jerome Singer:

> It is generally believed that it's good for you to see things or to imagine violent actions: the so-called catharsis theory that's still rife among some psychologists and certainly amongst a lot of literary types and people who produce television shows. And they really believe it's good for children to see all kinds of violence or good for adults to watch prizefighting and shooting and all sorts of things, because you get rid of that burbling inner aggression that you have.
>
> All the evidence we have in psychology suggests the contrary. The more you watch aggressive material, the more likely you are to be aggressive.

Another major concern about the effects of excessive TV viewing is the impact on young people's development of imagination. Jerome

Singer, director of the Graduate Program in Clinical Psychology at Yale University and codirector of the Family Television Research and Consulting Center, has done extensive research on the origins of daydreams in children's make-believe and fantasy activity. Many of the studies have specifically investigated the role of TV, because nowadays, just as we get all kinds of things in packages, we also get packaged fantasies: just flip on a TV set. One might think that watching a lot of TV would stimulate creativity, because after all, programming is so imaginative, isn't it?

Heavy viewing of TV among children actually seems to be associated with less imagination, partly because fancy is to some extent developed through practice. Kids may sit on the floor, take two blocks, and then put them together, making a little game. This type of activity is critical. But if kids don't have time to play, because they're watching so much TV, when *do* they get to practice imagination?

Such data are particularly alarming when we consider that the average preschooler spends about four hours a day watching television—and that viewing time increases as children get older. Overall, children spend more time watching television than they do attending school!

Getting involved in positive social change at some level, however modest—from fixing a broken window to challenging irresponsible television programming (or, better yet, curbing excessive TV viewing)—may seem far afield from traditional notions of health education and promotion. But the process of environmental intervention is a logical extension of the drive to nurture, which is where we began; keeping alive the creative promise for ourselves and our children involves not only raising them to be healthy but providing them with a healthy environment in which to live and thrive. Still, environmental intervention doesn't have to be dramatic in order to be profound. Sometimes the simplest ideas can revive the sense of wonder we seek.

Consider the innovative example of the Sky Awareness Project, the brainchild of Jack Borden, a retired Boston newscaster. During a hike ten years ago, Borden was struck by the "beauty, majesty, and fragility" of the sky. He decided to approach local schools with the idea of using the sky to stimulate learning. After founding a non-profit organization called For Spacious Skies, he issued a thirty-two-page guide for teachers. Since then, a variety of stimulating programs have been incorporated in Borden's idea: participants listen to "sky music," write cloud-inspired haiku, and use star charts to locate constellations. Best of all, the sky is free, and generously bestows its beauty on inner-city students as well as children living in the country. According to Harvard Graduate School researchers, the emphasis on looking up, followed by drawing pictures and writing about the sky, significantly increased the level of aesthetic sensitivity among participants, particularly in the areas of visual art and literature. Said one instructor, "I've been teaching school for twenty-three years, and I've never seen anything sustain children's learning and aesthetic appreciation like this program. It is a complete curriculum that addresses every subject and competency area with meaning."

The Sky Awareness Project is a great stimulus for environmental concern because children explore sky-related subjects such as astronomy, meteorology, and agriculture. Everyone is affected. After one sunrise celebration, teachers received the following note: "I am sixty-five years old, and this is the first time I have seen a sunrise. I'm here with my grandchild. Thank you."

3

The Chemical Brain

Molecules and Mood

The astonishing hypothesis is that you, your joys, and your sorrows, your memories and ambitions, your sense of personal identity and free will, are in fact no more than the behavior of a vast assembly of nerve cells and their associated molecules. As Lewis Carroll's Alice might have phrased it, "You're nothing but a pack of neurons."

—Francis H. C. Crick

The Language of the Brain

"The language of the brain is chemistry," Avram Goldstein declared in 1982. This assertion rings louder and truer with each passing year; scarcely a week goes by without a dramatic revelation in scientific circles regarding the influence that the chemistry of the brain exerts over our thoughts, moods, and actions. In recognition of the mounting tide of brain research and its significance in understanding human behavior, the U.S. Congress has designated the 1990s as "The Decade of the Brain."

As our understanding grows, we are beginning to recognize that it may be possible to control the brain quite as much as it controls us. Indeed, we already have the ability to alter our behavior and mental processes by managing the chemistry of the brain itself. By gaining insight into how the brain works, we can make healthier choices about how to feel good and select those pathways to pleasure which result in optimal living.

In our seminars on the "Chemistry of Craving," we often encounter students who volunteer that they would never have taken this or that drug had they known how it may have affected their brains. For example, an understanding of brain chemistry enabled one student to choose the excitement of competitive sports rather than the risk of taking cocaine. He had come to realize that, while both activities produce heightened states of arousal, cocaine promised him an array of harmful consequences (including its effects on the brain's own "wiring"), whereas is participation in sports promoted his health and well-being.

Unfortunately, brain chemistry is rarely considered in discussions of human behavior and the mysteries of personality. Personality is believed to be the product of genetics and environment: genes set the predisposition; family and culture guide how we ultimately think, act, and feel. Chemistry is . . . well, it's one of the hard sciences, isn't it? It has something to do with molecules, right? The language of the brain might be chemistry, but for most of us, it's a foreign language, a bizarre shorthand of letters interspersed with numbers: H_2O, $C_6H_{12}O_6$, CH_3CH_2OH.

Let's put aside the shorthand for a moment and talk about the substances themselves. On an elemental level (no pun intended), they are largely responsible for who you are. Without water (H_2O), you would become dehydrated, like a parched autumn leaf, and perish. Without glucose ($C_6H_{12}O_6$), a type of sugar, your body could not carry out any of its energy-dependent activities; the brain burns glucose as a stove burns wood. When alcohol (CH_3CH_2OH) is consumed and broken down, a powerful narcotic, abbreviated as THIQ, is formed. THIQ accounts for some of the strange behavior exhibited by people stumbling out of bars around closing time.

Chemical processes are at work in many of our deepest urges and predilections, from a child's preference for sweets to the smoker's craving for a cigarette. Even sexual behavior has a distinct chemical component. Special odors, called pheromones, carried through the skin as chemical attractants, are sexual invitations in humans and many other species. Whether we are aware of it or not, we are all driven by chemistry, like the male moth in Lewis Thomas's humorous essay "Fear of Pheromones":

The messages are urgent, but they may arrive, for all we know, in a fragrance of ambiguity. "At home, 4 p.m. today," says the female moth, and releases a brief explosion of bombykol, a single molecule of which will tremble the hairs of any male within miles and send him driving upwind in a confusion of ardor. But it is doubtful if he has an awareness of being caught in an aerosol of chemical attractant. On the contrary, he probably finds suddenly that it has become an excellent day, the weather remarkably bracing, the time appropriate for a bit of exercise of the old wings, a brisk turn upward. En route, traveling the gradient of bombykol, he notes the presence of other males, heading in the same direction, all in a good mood, inclined to race for the sheer sport of it. Then, when he reaches his destination, it may seem to him the most extraordinary, the greatest piece of luck: "Bless my soul, what have we here!"

While the relationship between chemistry and behavior is vast and intricate, for now we need only focus on those functions of brain chemistry which have been most directly linked to mood. The brain, "the soul's frail dwelling place," is actually a giant pharmaceutical factory manufacturing a myriad of different molecules, each exerting its own effect on our emotional state. Figure 3.1 illustrates the relationship between molecules and mood.

Molecules known as neurotransmitters (lower left), released from one nerve cell (neuron), activate another neuron that is part of a larger neuronal network, such as the limbic system. If enough of the neurons in this network are activated, higher centers in the brain interpret the signals from this network as joy, sorrow, anger, or some other conscious emotional state. Depending on the molecules generated, the resulting mood can range from the extreme torment of depression to the most intense thrill of ecstasy. Those molecules generated within our brains which have the greatest effect on our emotions are known as neurotransmitters. Neurotransmitters may be produced as a result of various mental or physical activities: listening to music, finding beauty in nature or art, having physical contact with another person, engaging in sexual activity, savoring moments of intense nostalgia—to name just a few.

We have a tendency to romanticize our emotional states, of course—to regard them as something largely out of our control and even outside of ourselves, as when we talk of being "swept away" with passion, "seized" by anger, or "transported" by a song. Yet it is also possible to evoke neuronal responses by artificial means. For example, powerful drugs such as cocaine and heroin, when injected, smoked, snorted, or whatever, can mimic the effect of these natural

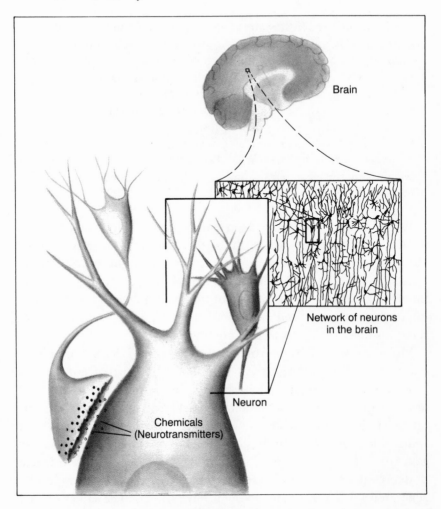

FIGURE 3.1
Neuronal Pathways: From Molecules to Mood

molecules and evoke sensations of altered consciousness that the user interprets as pleasurable. In fact, many people utilize the effect of these drugs on the brain to titrate their mood, much as a chemist regulates the acidity of a solution by adding a little base, then a little acid, then a little more base to achieve the desired result. As we shall see, it is also possible to regulate our emotional states by nondrug activities that alter the amount of neurotransmitters in the brain.

The production of these molecules is a complex chemical process that scientists are still struggling to explain. Although the metaphor is often taken too literally, it is helpful to consider the brain as an electrochemical computer as well as a chemical factory. Its 100 billion or so nerve cells are able to store more information than all the libraries in the world combined. Each of these neurons is in turn composed of three basic elements (Figure 3.2).

The nucleus of the cell (soma) constitutes a miniature brain within a larger brain. It is the soma that "decides" to transmit a message (actually, a particular kind of electrical impulse) from one nerve cell to the next, or to ignore it. This is the only decision the soma needs to make, but it must make that decision very quickly. Like a computer, the soma is "a fast idiot," following commands and unable to make judgments. Connected to the soma is a long fiber, the axon, through which the message must travel on its way to the next neuron. The message is transferred from one of the many branches at the end of the axon of the sending neuron to one of a number of

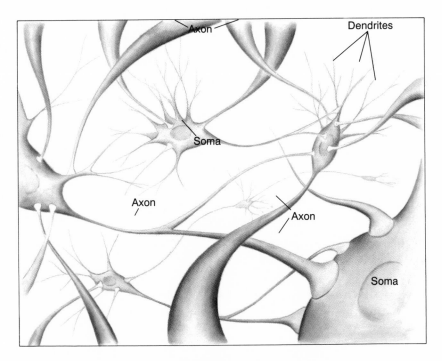

FIGURE 3.2
Neurons: The Brain's Electrochemical Hardware

branches on the receiving cell. These branches are called dendrites; each neuron may have up to 10,000 dendrites. If we consider the possibilities of interaction between the 100 billion neurons found in the human brain with 10,000 dendrites per neuron, we have the possibility of quadrillions of connections—different ways to send messages to different "receivers," with different results. This makes the brain the most complex entity in the universe.

Incredibly, this process of communication between neuron and neuron is carried out without any direct physical contact between the two cells—as if this were all taking place in a city of trillions of people, all talking to each other on cellular telephones! Neurons are separated by a gap known as the synapse or synaptic junction. Chemical changes that occur in these neuronal spaces determine how we respond to each "message"; this process of communication between neurons, known as neurotransmission, is largely responsible for the brain functions that determine our individual personalities, intellect, and character. It is precisely because the neurons are separated by a synapse—in other words, they are not "hardwired"—that the brain ends up with nearly limitless options for neurotransmission.

This state of affairs is both good news and bad news. The good news is that neurochemical options are what enable us to utilize our brain to find pathways to pleasure; but the bad news is that this opportunity for exploring endless variations of neurotransmission also permits us to fashion living hells for ourselves and those around us.

Obviously, the neurotransmitters responsible for carrying vital messages from neuron to neuron—messages registering pain, euphoria, fear, excitement—must be truly remarkable chemicals, the "wonder drugs" of the entire central nervous system. Consider, for example, the astonishing effects of norepinephrine (NE), a neurotransmitter found in that part of the brain known as the locus coeruleus (Fig. 3.3).

One of NE's primary functions is to produce arousal and excitability, including the "fight or flight" phenomenon associated with the release of adrenaline. To understand how NE operates, it is helpful to start with a real-life situation.

Suppose you come home late, dog-tired from working the swingshift and barely able to stay awake long enough to unlock

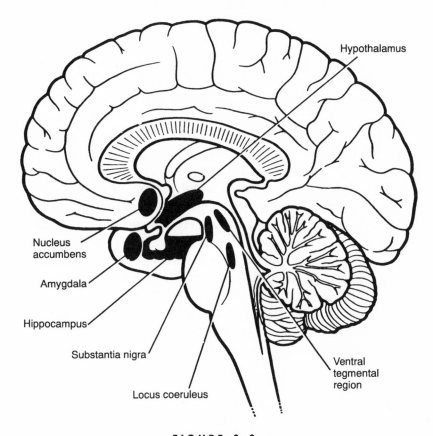

FIGURE 3.3

*Cross-Section of the Brain Showing Major Components
of the Limbic System*

Source: Adapted from Blum, K. (1991). Alcohol and the Addictive Brain:
New Hope for Alcoholics from Biogenetic Research. New York:
Macmillan.

your door. Your brain appears to be almost nonfunctional, unable
to perform the simplest task, such as taking off your shoes. You unlock the door, turn on the light, and shuffle toward the bedroom.
Suddenly, the bathroom door at the other end of the house flies open
and out comes a wild-eyed intruder, so fierce in appearance that he
makes Charles Manson look like Dick Clark. He starts toward you,
waving a knife with a six-inch blade. In this instant, all drowsiness
vanishes. Your brain is suddenly racing at full throttle.

You judge the attacker's forward speed while simultaneously
scanning the room for a weapon to protect yourself. Out of the cor-

ner of your eye, you spot the very heavy bronze statue of Lord Shiva brought back from India last year. Although the statue is ordinarily far too heavy to use as a weapon, you grab it with one hand and raise it above your head as if it were a police officer's billy club. The intruder, seeing himself in mortal danger, veers aside and races out the door. The danger has passed; but two hours later, you're still wide awake and unable to sleep.

What happened? What transformed you from a half-awake zombie into an alert, highly tuned fighting machine? The answer has to do with a split-second electrochemical process in your brain—although it's going to take a little longer than that to explain. As the intruder rushes towards you, the dangerous image suddenly looming in your half-conscious vision signals brain chemistry to spring into action. This action is illustrated in Figure 3.4, indicating what occurs at a single synaptic junction between two neurons during this episode:

Chemical messages flow from the axon on the left (presynaptic) neuron across the synapse to the dendrite of the postsynaptic neuron on the right and then on to the soma of the same neuron. As the impulse reaches the presynaptic terminal, specific channels open in the membrane of this neuron. This allows doubly charged calcium atoms (ions) to enter the cell, which in turn stimulates the release of the neurotransmitter—in this case, NE (illustrated by diamond-shaped molecules)—into the synapse. NE moves across the synapse, carrying the message to the postsynaptic neuron. Embedded in the outer membrane of this neuron are complex chemicals that act as receptors for NE. These receptors have specific shapes that exactly complement the shape of NE. This enables the molecules of NE to attach themselves to these receptors in much the same way that a key fits a lock. In fact, the key must not only fit the lock but also open the door; just as many Cadillac keys will fit the locks of Buicks but will not open the doors, the same is true of neurotransmitters and receptors.

Fortunately for you, when you surprise the burglar, norepinephrine not only fits the locks but opens the doors (ion channels) of the cell. Opening the cell doors allows certain ions (potassium, sodium, and chloride) to go in and out of this cell. If enough channels are opened and enough ions go in and out, the electrical nature of the cell's outer membrane is altered (depolarized). This enables the mes-

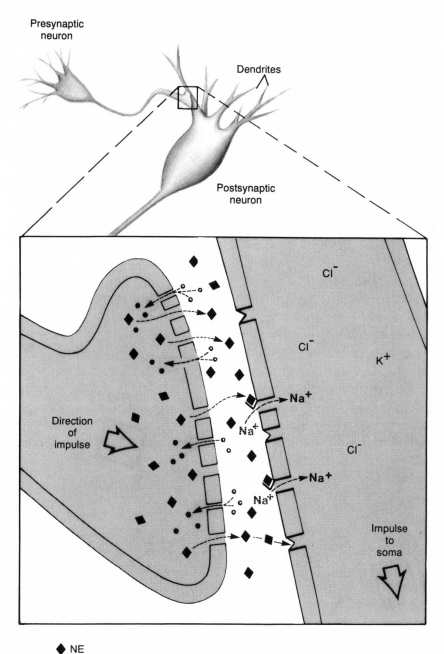

FIGURE 3.4
The Synaptic Junction and Chemical Transmission

sage to be sent to the soma of the postsynaptic cell, where it is processed with input from thousands of other cells, all undergoing the same process.

Before the membrane of the postsynaptic cell can "fire" (become depolarized and send its impulse to the soma), a critical number of receptor sites must be occupied by NE. The more molecules of this neurotransmitter that we can shove into the synapse, the quicker this critical number of sites will be occupied. Imagine trying to fill the holes of an egg carton by dropping Ping-Pong balls from ten feet. Many of the balls will not land in the holes of the egg carton; if we want to fill the carton quickly, we need to drop more Ping-Pong balls in a given period of time. In the case of neurotransmission, the more molecules of NE released into the synapse, the sooner these receptor sites are occupied—and the more rapidly the neurons will fire.

Now let's go back to that burglar. As you stumble toward the door, half-asleep, the presynaptic neuron is releasing NE at a very slow rate. Slow neurotransmission in NE neuronal pathways is manifested as drowsiness and mental lethargy. If someone asked you at this time to solve a simple math problem or lift the statue of Lord Shiva with one hand, you could do neither. Suddenly, the intruder appears from behind the bathroom door, obviously bent on causing you serious bodily harm. Your brain comes to the rescue. The presynaptic neuron opens its channels and floods the synapse with NE, which quickly attaches itself to receptors on the postsynaptic membrane. Within a split second, enough receptors are occupied to depolarize this membrane and cause it to fire. The receptors quickly dump the NE back into the synapse. This allows the membrane to repolarize, preparing the receptors to receive more NE, which the presynaptic terminals now release at an "alarming" rate. In a very short time, the neuron fires another and yet another impulse. Thanks to the abrupt surge in neurotransmission, your mood suddenly swings from somber to frightened, preparing you to face the burglar or run.

Simultaneously, electrical impulses race forward along pathways from the locus coeruleus to higher brain centers, increasing your alertness and cognitive ability. This, among other mental changes, helps you to gauge the speed of the intruder while simultaneously searching for a weapon. The process also signals the hypothalamus to send messages to the pituitary gland, which in turn causes the adrenal cortex to produce adrenaline. The activation of this system, known as the HPA axis, accelerates the heart rate, bringing oxygen and other nutrients to the various parts of the body, increasing strength, and decreasing reflex time. Following the departure of the intruder, you are unable to sleep for many hours, because the chemicals (NE) produced by this episode cascade back and forth across the synapse, keeping the rate of neurotransmission high, your eyes wide awake, and your brain pulsating.

What makes neurotransmission so remarkable is the speed with which this seemingly very cumbersome and complex process occurs. It is like running a marathon race in which there are a thousand streams to cross. At each stream, the runner must gather rocks (neurotransmitters) from the first shore (presynaptic terminal) to build stepping-stones to the next shore (postsynaptic terminal). The encounter with the intruder increases the number of "neuronal" rocks that are available on the shore where the runner arrives (presynaptic neuron); the more rocks available, the more rapidly will the runner be able to build a path to cross over the stream.

Of course, most activities in which we engage do not alter our consciousness to the level of arousal brought on by the attack of the burglar. Although this increase in neurotransmission is brought about without the use of drugs, it would be misleading to classify this experience as a natural high. Clearly, the accelerated brain chemistry involved in this incident would not lead to optimization of lifelong pleasures, especially if experienced on a continuing basis. The burglar scenario should, however, give you some idea of how the mind and body can be energized, how mood can dramatically shift, and how the moment can be seized—all through the power of brain chemistry. We may not be able (or want) to induce such an intense state of alarm, yet we can invoke more pleasant and controllable emotional states on our own.

Arousal Junkies

There are many avenues we can take to control our brain chemistry. The particular avenue we choose is highly dependent on our individual personalities. C. R. Cloninger of Washington University in St. Louis has classified personality types into three main categories: novelty-seeking, harm avoidance, and reward dependence.

These broad categories are analogous to the categories of arousal, relaxation, and fantasy that we proposed in 1983. For those ecstasy junkies at the top end of the scale—Cloninger's novelty-seekers—nothing less than the frenetic popping and cracking of their neurons will satisfy their need for instant gratification.

Cloninger notes that those who rate moderately high on his novelty-seeking scale "usually seek exhilaration from thrilling adventures and exploration of unfamiliar places and situations." Calvin in "Calvin & Hobbes" (1992) embodies this quest in its most primal form, as he and Hobbes once again careen wildly down a steep, snow-covered slope on their trusty sled:

> If you ask me, Hobbes, the whole notion of "instant gratification" is a myth!
>> I don't ever get what I want when I want it! I always have to wait!
>> Look how long it's taken me to be six years old! Practically forever!

The sled zooms off a snowbank as Calvin exclaims:

> When do I get to drive? When can I go see gory, violent movies?! Why do I have to wait till I'm older?

The sled manages to stay upright and finally nears the bottom of the hill, with Calvin growing ever more impatient. As the sled gains momentum, so does Calvin:

> People say life's a journey, but I'm tired of wasting my precious time in transit! I say, if you want to find out where the road goes, get in the fast lane and hit the gas!

The sled slams into a rock. Calvin and Hobbes are thrown off. As they are tumbling through the air, Calvin shouts:

> Spare me the scenery and let's get where we're going! I'm a busy guy! I've got places to be!

The two of them crawl out of the snow, and Calvin utters a profound truism that could serve as a reminder to all those who prefer life in the fast lane:

Gosh, that was over quick.

But true arousal junkies tend not to be dissuaded by the risks or the impermanence of their sensation-seeking. Regardless of whether one is traveling by sled, drugs, or some other means of conveyance, the allure of this mad dash to unexplored terrain remains the same. It has to do with the chemical changes that occur in the brain's own "fast lane."

One very windy day in the spring of 1987, one of us (Sunderwirth) was driving south out of San Francisco when he noticed several hang gliders diving and swooping over the dunes near the ocean. He stopped the car and walked over to get a closer look at the action.

What an incredible sight! The takeoff point was a high dune with an updraft on the steep side. The pilots would carry their gliders up the side of the dune opposite the updraft; once at the top, they would strap on their harness and dive headlong into the wind. Sometimes it seemed as if they might crash into the sandy beach before becoming safely airborne. Once they caught the wind, however, they would soar high above the earth like giant multicolored hawks, occasionally swooping dangerously close to the ground, as if they were diving for some unseen prey.

The author watched one particularly adventuresome glider pilot, who constantly took what seemed to be extremely high risks, guiding her craft into dives that brought her to within a few feet of the sand. Once she was safely on the ground, he engaged her in conversation, hoping to gain some insight into her emotional state as she played her private game of "chicken" with the wind and the sea. Asked how she felt about gambling with injury or death, she replied without hesitation, "It's better than an orgasm."

It's not uncommon for hang-gliding enthusiasts to liken their experience to the intense pleasure of sexual release. (The same can be said for surfers, sky divers, bungee jumpers, etc.) An adrenaline rush does have its pleasurable aspects—even though it's primarily a signal of danger. In fact, the rapid influx of neurotransmitters into the synapse during a hang-gliding flight is not unlike that which occurred in the episode involving the burglar. This self-induced increase in neurotransmission produced by high-risk activities is what we have called "the joy of fear." And as with any powerful jolt to the system, whether it comes from drugs or risk-taking, the subject can come to depend on the frenzied neuronal firing for pleasure and feel the pangs of withdrawal when the sensation can no longer be obtained.

"What happens," our adrenaline junkie was asked, "if you are not able to fly for long periods of time?" She replied:

> Once I broke my leg attempting a really stupid maneuver. For a number of weeks, I was not able to fly. I've never been so depressed in my life. Nothing seemed to interest me. I just sat around, waiting for the day I could start flying again.

For some people, hang gliding is a perfectly acceptable way to achieve a neurochemical rush, one that makes many other kinds of physical activity seem pallid and boring. What many of us may find "wild" or even suicidal, the true enthusiasts may regard as poetic, orgasmic, perhaps spiritual in its intensity.

Yet this hunger for ecstasy has its dark side. It can be particularly disturbing when it finds expression in activities far more dangerous than hang gliding, activities associated with compulsive, deviant, and even violent behavior. There are criminals who talk about the joy of fear, too; but they're talking about a kind of ecstasy that comes from fantasizing about, and acting out, "extreme" behavior—behavior that can be compulsive, possibly addictive, as the subject comes to rely on the chemical changes involved to meet some dark need of his or her own. Ronald is a convicted rapist who has spent twenty-five years in prison and was sentenced to but did not serve two life sentences in hospitals for the criminally insane. He describes himself as a "habitual criminal" the way another man might describe himself as a drug addict. It's his entire identity:

> It is the ecstasy caused by fear that is addicting, not the actual act of rape. Prowling the neighborhood, skulking in shadows, dressing in black, wearing a ski mask, carrying a knife, breaking into the house: these are what I craved. The habitual criminal has turned fear into pleasure. Even the fantasy involved in planning the next crime is an unbelievable high. I would get such a euphoria from fantasizing that I was unable to function in a job; I would even get so aroused that I became psychotic as thoughts poured into my brain almost too fast to comprehend. Then the crime itself would create such an additional adrenaline rush that I could hardly remember the actual criminal act.

You can be certain of one thing: it's not the orgasm of the sex act that drove me—that was only the icing on the cake. The ecstasy of crime is the fear, and it's free.

The addictive nature of the excitement of crime is a theme that surfaces in many cases of career criminals, from pattern rapists to home invaders and even serial killers such as Jeffrey Dahmer, whose grim executions included elements of necrophilia and cannibalism. Detective Dennis Murphy, who interviewed Dahmer, testified at his sanity trial:

He [Dahmer] felt fright for fear of being caught, and excitement for knowing what he had done. . . . He stated that every time he would try to overcome his feelings of wanting to kill and dismember people, they would haunt him and overcome him just like an addiction.

Jumpstarting Pleasure

From self-induced, potentially life-threatening activities to substance abuse is but a small neurochemical step. For the arousal-prone or "novelty-seeking" person, stimulant drugs such as cocaine, amphetamine, speed, and ephedrine can hold tremendous appeal because they mimic the alterations in brain chemistry brought about by risk-taking activities. The "rush" experienced by the cocaine user is produced through an increase in the number of excitatory neurotransmitters in the synaptic junctions between neurons, which is translated into a corresponding acceleration in the rate of neuronal firing.

To understand this action, let's return briefly to our discussion of "normal" (drug-free) neurotransmission. In the absence of cocaine, excitatory neurotransmitters such as dopamine and norepinephrine are transported back and forth between the presynaptic and the postsynaptic neuron. After leaving the presynaptic neuron, crossing the synaptic junction, and attaching themselves to the receptors on the post-synaptic neuron, these neurotransmitters are then released back into the synapse, just as a key is removed from a lock. Here some of them will encounter a form of molecules called enzymes, which destroy them by crunching them into smaller molecules. Those which escape the jaws of these enzymes search for entrance doors in the wall of the presynaptic neuron; once safely inside, they

can be used again. These entrances are different from the exit holes
that allowed the neurotransmitters to leave the presynaptic neuron
in the first place.

Cocaine, acting like a palace guard, blocks these entrance doors,
preventing the neurotransmitters from reentering the presynaptic
neuron (Fig. 3.5).

At the same time, cocaine does not prevent neurotransmitters
from leaving this neuron. This results in the synapse becoming
crowded with neurotransmitters, faster than the enzymes can destroy them. This increased concentration of neurotransmitters al-

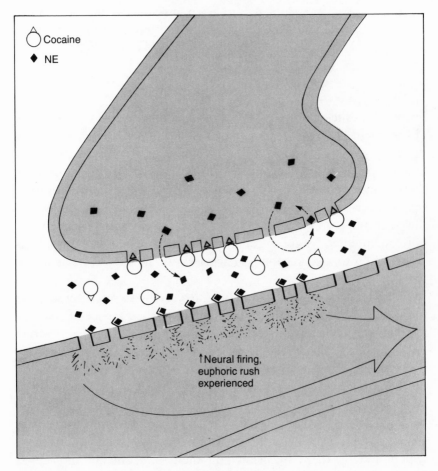

FIGURE 3.5
Cocaine in the Brain

lows more of the postsynaptic receptors to be occupied, resulting in an increase in neuronal firing, thereby creating the euphoric rush characteristic of cocaine (especially crack) use. In a sense, the brain has been tricked by this "chemical prostitute" into an "unnatural high," one with psychological and physiological effects similar to those produced by the attack of the burglar, the flight of the hang glider, and the skulking of the rapist. The brain doesn't distinguish clearly between a synaptic increase in excitatory neurotransmitters brought on by blocking the removal of these molecules from the synapse (cocaine) and an increase caused by pushing more of these neurotransmitters into the synapse (burglar-bashing); indeed, some drugs, such as amphetamine and speed, mimic the burglar-bashing scenario by enhancing the release of excitatory neurotransmitters from the presynaptic neuron into the synapse, thereby creating an excess of these molecules in the synapse. Either process results in a state of synthetic euphoria that can be perceived as exciting, disturbing, better than an orgasm—at first.

Obviously, this kind of dramatic rise in the rate of excitatory neurotransmission—whether through drugs, hang gliding, or crime—isn't the kind of high we refer to as natural, or the sort of life-fulfilling activities described by Robert Ornstein and David Sobel in their appropriately titled book *Healthy Pleasures*. These euphorias may very easily lead to a dysfunctional lifestyle characterized by compulsion, continuation, and harmful consequences. The individual who seeks pleasure through exhilaration and arousal must discover those activities which can bring about fulfillment and lifelong satisfaction without the hidden but all-too-common curse of addiction. As we shall see in subsequent chapters, pursuing such activities involves making a basic choice to seek prolonged pleasure rather than sustained ecstasy. Chemically speaking, pleasure is no problem; but the attempts to capture and sustain ecstasy are bound to fail.

Life in Cruise Control

Obviously, not everyone is a Type A individual, seeking arousal or stimulation as the primary means of enhancing feelings of well-being and decreasing anxiety. Many people seek pleasure by engaging in activities that produce a more relaxed and tranquil emotional state: meditation, for example, or watching television, listening to music, or sedating themselves with drugs or food. An extreme and obviously ridiculous example of this is the role that television often plays in "Calvin & Hobbes." Sometimes, it seems, our friend Calvin is inclined to see himself as a relaxation-prone (and we do mean prone) individual, rather than as a fearlessly sledding explorer.

In one episode, as Calvin turns on the TV, he proclaims his dislike for adventure:

I try to make television-watching a complete forfeiture of experience.

He then slouches in order to minimize expenditure of energy.

Notice how I keep my jaw slack, so my mouth hangs open. I try not to swallow either, so I drool, and I keep my eyes half-focused so I don't use any muscles at all.

His self-imposed lethargy then extends to his entire body.

I take a passive entertainment and extend the passivity to my entire being. I wallow in my lack of participation and response. I'm utterly inert.

As Hobbes leaves in disgust, Calvin proclaims,

I can almost feel my neural transmitters shutting down.

We often ask our audiences how many of them prefer relaxation, rather than arousal or fantasy, as their primary means of seeking pleasure. Surprisingly, the audiences often are divided equally among these three choices. In other words, two-thirds of us have no interest in skydiving, hang gliding, or bungee jumping. We're uncomfortable with neurotransmission in overdrive; we don't want to "seize the day"—we'd rather make it let go of us.

But does that necessarily make us passive couch potatoes, deprived of all sensation, our neural transmitters all shut down? Not at all. Just as the brain can produce molecules to stimulate and excite, it can also generate pleasure by producing appropriate molecules through relaxation- and satiation-oriented activities.

One of the brain's mysterious neurotransmitters is serotonin—which, as we mentioned earlier, is released into the brain by Grandmother's remedy of milk and cookies at bedtime and brings about the relaxation necessary for sleep. Serotonin's action, however, is much more complicated than Grandmother realized. In fact, it's so complex that there are now an average of four scientific articles published every day, seven days a week, attempting to determine the effect of serotonin on our mind, mood, and behavior.

Our discussion of serotonin's effects, like our description of brain chemistry in general, must necessarily be extremely simplified. We have no intention of attempting to explain the myriad of nearly incomprehensible chemical reactions occurring in the brain that contribute to our emotional states as well as to our very personalities. A detailed description of neurochemistry is beyond the purpose of this book, and in any case, scientific understanding of brain chemistry remains tentative, despite the thousands of articles published every month.

What is known about serotonin, though, suggests that it interacts with the brain in a number of ways, one of which is to stimulate release of opiate-like compounds known as endorphins and enkephalins. These compounds, in turn, behave in many ways like opiate drugs, such as morphine or heroin, to create a sense of euphoria and well-being.

One group of endorphins and enkephalins, discovered by Hughes and Kosterlitz in 1974, seems to play a prominent role in the pleasure generated by certain relaxation activities. The prominent neuroscientist Ken Blum of the University of Texas believes that release of these internal opioids brings about an indirect increase of the neurotransmitter dopamine in that region of the brain's reward system known as the nucleus accumbens (Fig. 3.3).

Understanding of the process by which the brain registers sensations of pleasure is far from complete. Much as we may think we know, the brain may indefinitely defy our attempts to unambiguously correlate a specific neurochemical process with a particular mood. But research on serotonin has provided us with one kind of model that helps us to follow what's going on in the brain that makes us feel so good.

Neurochemical Pleasure: The Keys to Paradise

Understanding of the feelings of pleasure evoked by brain chemistry properly begins with a search for a site in the brain responsible for this pleasure. The presence of a "pleasure center" in the brain was demonstrated by James Olds and Peter Milner at McGill University in the 1950s. They found that a rat with an electrode implanted into a certain region of the brain would continually press a lever in order to receive electrical stimulation. Aryeh Routtenberg of Northwestern University later showed that, given a choice between a lever that delivered food for survival and one delivering brain stimulation, rats would forgo food in favor of the "reward" of brain stimulation. In other words, they chose ecstasy over survival. Rats, it seems, may become as addicted to an artificial (and ultimately fatal) paradise as humans.

In these experiments, the preference for "prolonged ecstasy" occurred only if the electrode was placed in a very small part of the brain, which Routtenberg referred to as the "Reward Center." In recent years, the search for the specific site in the brain that regulates mood has led scientists to a complex array of neuronal clusters known as the limbic system. This region of the brain is believed to control emotions and is often referred to as the "reptilian brain," since we share this primordial brain with other living creatures.

Ken Blum has proposed a model for reward (pleasure) involving the interaction of several neurotransmitters with the various parts of the limbic system that compose the reward center. Blum proposes that the release of dopamine into the nucleus accumbens (Fig. 3.3), an important reward site, plays a major role in mediating our moods. (Although there are other reward sites in the limbic system, for simplicity we will limit our discussion to the action of dopamine on the nucleus accumbens.) In Blum's model, which he calls the "Reward Cascade," feelings of well-being, as well as the absence of craving and anxiety, depend on an adequate supply of dopamine to the nucleus accumbens. Any deficiency or imbalance that would lead to a deficit of dopamine would produce anxiety and a craving for substances (alcohol, cocaine, etc.) or activities involving risk-taking (gambling, crime, and even hang gliding) that would temporarily restore this deficit.

Figure 3.6 helps us to understand this complex interaction of neurotransmitters. Let's start with serotonin, that ubiquitous neurotransmitter about which thousands of articles have been written. In the hypothalamus, serotonin neurons stimulate the release of methi-

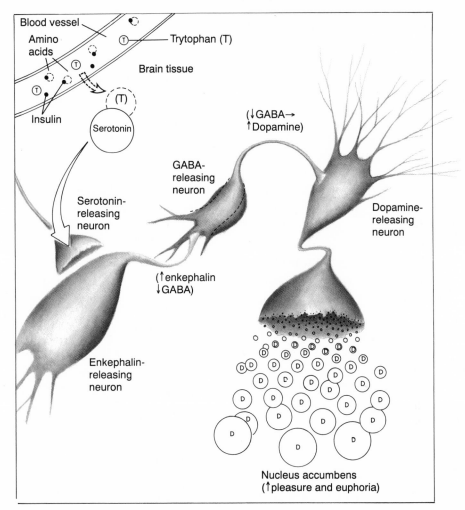

FIGURE 3.6
The Reward Cascade of the Human Brain

onine enkephalin, which in turn inhibits the release of GABA (gamma aminobutyric acid) in the limbic system.

What is GABA? In our previous discussion of neurotransmission, we limited our remarks to excitatory pathways, whose neurotransmitters enhance neurotransmission and therefore create elevated emotional states. The brain must also have other pathways that retard excitatory neurotransmission; otherwise, we would be in a constant state of emotional turmoil. GABA is the neurotransmitter utilized by these inhibitory synapses; it's our own internal "Valium," regulating our mood through inhibition of the release of dopamine to the nucleus accumbens.

Now that we have struggled through these technical terms, let's see what they really mean in terms of our emotional state. As we retrace the Reward Cascade, keep in mind that an adequate supply of dopamine and therefore dopamine neurotransmission in the nucleus accumbens is necessary for feelings of well-being. We have seen that increased neurotransmission in the nucleus accumbens can lead to excitation and arousal; now let's see how increased neurotransmission can have the effect of decreasing anxiety, too.

Remember Grandmother's milk and cookies? Milk contains the amino acid tryptophan, which, when it reaches the brain, is converted into that miracle neurotransmitter serotonin. Sounds simple enough: just drink milk, relax, and go to sleep. But like everything else in brain chemistry and in life, it's not that simple. The complication is that tryptophan, from milk or any other source, does not compete well with other amino acids in getting from the blood into the brain. There is a barrier that restricts the entrance of many chemicals trying to get into the brain from the blood. This barrier, which acts like a snooty doorman at a fashionable nightclub, will allow only certain molecules to enter. The barrier serves a critical function in keeping poisons out of the brain; but unfortunately, for some reason it apparently fails to recognize the importance of serotonin.

That's where the cookies come in. If your grandmother's cookies are like ours, they contain large amounts of both simple carbohydrates (table sugar) and complex carbohydrates (starch). These stimulate the release of insulin, the chemical secreted by the pancreas to metabolize sugar. But the insulin doesn't just go to work on the carbohydrates; it removes any of the other amino acids, except tryptophan, from the blood. (Tryptophan, unlike the other amino acids, has a protective coating that protects it from being affected by insulin.) This eases the competition in the bloodstream and allows tryptophan to slip past the blood-brain barrier (the doorman in our analogy) to enter the brain, where it is converted into the neurotransmitter serotonin.

So, now that we have a supply of serotonin, what does it do for us? How does it help us not only to sleep but in general to reduce feelings of anxiety and craving? In the hypothalamus (Fig. 3.3), serotonin-releasing neurons impinge on enkephalin neurons, enhancing their release. The primary function of enkephalin neurons in the brain is to inhibit the release of neurotransmitters from any neuron with which they interact; the more enkephalin released from these neurons, the more inhibition they exert (Fig. 3.6). Conveniently, GABA-releasing neurons, as well as other neurons, have receptor sites for enkephalin molecules. As the number of these receptor sites occupied with enkephalin molecules increases, the release of GABA decreases. But GABA, remember, keeps the release of dopamine in check through another inhibitory synapse; as GABA decreases, we can expect the release of dopamine to increase. In other words, the enkephalin has inhibited the inhibitor. This process works with the logic of a double negative and results in a positive increase in dopamine at the nucleus accumbens, which brings about a decrease in feelings of restlessness and anxiety. Serotonin (from milk and cookies) is the battery, allowing the brain to start the Reward Cascade ending in enhanced neurotransmission. Grandmother knew her neurochemistry!

Although serotonin will fire up the Reward Cascade, the real power behind the pleasure pathway is enkephalin, that internal opioid produced by our brains in response to both internal and external stimuli. It is this euphoric effect that has resulted in enkephalins and their cousins, the endorphins, being referred to as "The Keys to Paradise." Enkephalins and endorphins, although structurally different, are often grouped together under the generic name endogenous opioids.

Not only do endogenous opioids create a sense of euphoria and well-being, but, in a manner similar to opiates like morphine and heroin, they also have a strong analgesic effect. It is this analgesic effect that enables a severely injured person or animal to ignore the pain of the injury and to engage in a lifesaving activity of fight or flight brought about by the release of the neurotransmitter norepinephrine. Were this not the case, the injured person (or animal) would be so overcome with pain as to be unable to fight back or run away. For an excellent example of the interaction of endorphins (to reduce pain) and norepinephrine (to stimulate action and enhance strength), we can turn to Bernal Diaz's description of the attack by

Hernán Cortés on the Aztec capital of Tenochtitlán, now known as Mexico City. In his description of the battle, Diaz recorded that there were no noncombative casualties as a result of injuries to the outnumbered conquistadores. All of the Spanish were either fighting or dead, even if the injuries were so serious that death ultimately followed.

Much to our credit—and eternal regret—humankind has been able to manufacture drugs such as morphine and heroin, which have chemical structures similar to our own endorphins and can produce the desired feeling of euphoric satiation. During the American Civil War, morphine was virtually the only drug available that could ease the horrific pain of the wounded and maimed, but the survivors paid dearly for their relief, returning home as addicts. Countless opiate users have followed in their footsteps.

As in the case of cocaine, opiates mimic the function of natural brain processes—with an extra kick. Although the brain can hold more information than all the libraries in the world, individual neurons are not too bright and cannot clearly distinguish morphine from endogenous opioids. Morphine and other opiate molecules can occupy receptor sites on the GABA-releasing neurons ordinarily reserved for endorphins. This flooding of the receptors with "phony" molecules brings about instant euphoria. Unfortunately, the sensation is more intense than that which can be elicited by listening to music, watching a beautiful sunset, or cuddling a favorite pet; inevitably, some relaxation-seekers wind up trying to fast-forward their moods to euphoric states by ingesting these drugs, just as arousal junkies escalate their arousal states through using cocaine. And, of course, the most likely results of such self-medication are addiction and the accompanying dysfunctional lifestyle.

Addiction: The Curse of Ecstasy

He who binds to himself a joy
Doth the winged life destroy;
But he who kisses the joy as it flies
Lives in eternity's sun rise.

—*William Blake*

The brain's own response to jolts of powerful drugs resembles William Blake's delineation of healthy and unhealthy approaches to joy—the person who "binds" a joy tends to destroy the "winged life." But why must it be that way? Why can't humans experience sustained euphoria without addiction? Why can't we, like Calvin in the "Calvin & Hobbes" episode in the introduction to this book, live out our fantasy of perpetual bliss:

> I want my life to be one never ending ascension!—For me it's only going to be up and up!

The answer lies in the chemical processes we've been describing. Calvin's quest is neurochemically impossible. The old adage "What goes up must come down" was surely written for the person attempting a life of continued greater and greater ecstasy. The hard truth is that the brain does resist, and very successfully, unceasing attempts at neurochemical alterations.

This resistance is part of the key to the survival of the human race. Through eons of evolutionary struggle, the brain has developed neurochemical "feedback" mechanisms that work against long-term dramatic alterations in neurotransmission and the accompanying mood and personality disorders. Obviously, short-term and rapid changes in neurotransmission, such as those occurring on encountering a saber-toothed tiger, had to be allowed if we were to survive. But for the long haul, inconsistent and erratic behavior as a result of uncontrolled neurotransmission would not enhance survival of a member of the species (e.g., any early humans too depressed to go out and seek game for self and family would be unlikely to pass their genes on to future generations).

This resistance to dramatic and extended changes in neurotransmission is, to a large extent, the result of regulating the number of neurotransmitters in the synapse between the neurons. It should be obvious that the brain must have mechanisms not only to regulate neurotransmission but to restore it to some normative "baseline" level, once this level has become disrupted. After your encounter with the burglar, your neurotransmission, which is completely out of control, has left you with a pounding heart, increased metabolism, rapid breathing, and no chance of sleeping for several hours. As soon as the danger is over, the brain goes to work to restore baseline neurotransmission. Otherwise, you would remain in this state of intensified animation until your body and brain "burned out."

We refer to this resistance to change as "synaptic homeostasis." The mechanism by which the brain regulates as well as restores our neurotransmission (and therefore our moods) is a combination of enzymatic and other chemical changes. Sidney Cohen has pointed out that the receptors on the post-synaptic neuron exhibit a self-regulatory capacity, which enables them to alter their sensitivity to neurotransmitters during episodes of either excessive or minimal concentration of neurotransmitters in the synapse. After we engage in any activity, healthy or unhealthy, that increases the number of neurotransmitters in the synapse—hang gliding, cocaine snorting, gambling, burglar-bashing—the restoring ability of the brain goes into action to minimize the effect of this altered neurotransmitter level. The brain can also utilize these same chemical mechanisms to restore synaptic homeostasis following activities that decrease neurotransmission, such as heroin use.

How does all of this relate to the phenomenon of addiction? Mary Barnes's bout with cocaine addiction, discussed earlier, provides us with a clear picture of the drug user's journey to oblivion. In a real sense, drug users are flirting with Mother Nature—and, as we all know from a certain margarine commercial, "It's not smart to fool Mother Nature." You can do it for a while, but not for long. Reflect for a moment on Mary's first encounter with cocaine. On first using the drug, Mary experiences a rush so intense and pleasant that she, like so many other cocaine users, wants to reexperience it at will. When the effects of this first drug experience wear off, though, her neurotransmission returns almost to normal. Mary must then repeat the drug experience if she is to remain high.

After a few such episodes with cocaine, something unsettling begins to happen. The dosage that initially could elicit intense euphoria seems to be losing its punch, because Mary's brain, recognizing the continued attempts to upset synaptic homeostasis, has begun to counter those attempts. Changes within the postsynaptic neuron cause the neurotransmitters that are already in the synapse to be less effective in raising neurotransmission. These changes are associated with the molecular complex formed by attachment of the neurotransmitter to the postsynaptic receptor (Fig. 3.4). In particular, they involve a change in the production of the enzyme adenylate cyclase.

In the absence of cocaine or other mind-altering drugs or activity, the brain maintains a fairly constant level of adenylate cyclase as part of its molecular mechanism to preserve synaptic homeostasis. But when adenylate cyclase, which is normally inactive, comes into contact with the neurotransmitter/receptor complex, it is structurally altered into an active form. In this active form, it initiates a chain reaction that ultimately results in opening additional ion doors in the postsynaptic membrane. This additional influx of ions into the postsynaptic neuron enhances the overall depolarization of this neuron's membrane, a process that is necessary before it can transmit the pulse. This is precisely what happened when Mary first began to use cocaine: her synapses would fill up with neurotransmitters, creating an abnormally large number of neurotransmitter/receptor complexes in the postsynaptic membrane. These complexes in turn activated an increased number of adenylate cyclase molecules, opening more doors for ions to flow into the postsynaptic neuron. This increased flow of ions then caused an increased rate of depolarization of the membrane, creating an abnormally rapid rate of neurotransmission—just what Mary wanted. But regardless of what Mary wants, the brain will not for long tolerate this artificially induced increase in the rate of neurotransmission.

One way to slow it down is to stop producing molecules of adenylate cyclase. This is accomplished through the brain's feedback mechanism, which signals the adenylate cyclase factory that too much of this enzyme is already present in the postsynaptic neuron. As the number of enzyme molecules decreases, those reactions which depend on this enzyme to get started are slowed down.

To make matters worse, the receptors on the postsynaptic neuron become less effective in producing neurotransmission. The brain has now become tolerant to the level of cocaine that Mary is used to ingesting. To reach the level of euphoria previously experienced, the amount of the drug must be increased. Soon this, too, fails to bring on the previous "high," as the brain responds by further increasing its own defenses against synaptic insult. The spiral of increased usage and diminishing results continues until you can get "normal" but you can't get "high." Unless one stops now, one could easily end up in the hospital, as Mary did—or in the morgue.

Why, then, is it so hard to stop? Because at some point in the process, the user has become dependent on the drug to prevent feelings of extreme dysphoria and is truly addicted. Mary has been using cocaine to fool her brain into rapid production of neurotransmitters—but then the brain's own biofeedback mechanisms step in to halt, or at least dramatically reduce, production of these neurotransmitters. Now the brain is primarily relying on exogenous chemicals to furnish the excitatory stimulus. When cocaine use is eliminated, there is now a shortage rather than a surplus of neurotransmitters in the synapse. This results in a reduction of neurotransmission to a level far below the baseline level prior to drug use. This failure to return neurotransmission to a baseline level is experienced as a "crash," leaving the abstinent addict with a greater craving for ecstasy than that experienced before drug use. Unfortunately, the baseline level of neurotransmission is not immediately restored, since it takes time to reverse the enzymatic and receptor changes brought on by drug use and to start up the neurotransmitter and enzyme factories again.

The brain also recognizes when a user attempts to alter neurotransmission by using opiates. Opiates such as heroin and morphine upset synaptic homeostasis by initially altering neurotransmission in certain parts of the limbic system, as well as in the pain pathways. The addiction process is similar to what we've been describing with cocaine: an opiate such as heroin displaces our own natural endorphins from their receptor sites and creates an artificial euphoria of instant and intense bliss. But this chemical paradise has a short life, and another fix is soon required to maintain the desired level of hedonic intensity. Once again, Mother Nature is not going to sit idly by; she will use the same basic chemical alterations used to thwart the cocaine user. In this instance, that means dramatically altering the enzymatic levels in that part of the Reward Cascade responsible for releasing dopamine into the nucleus accumbens. This drug-induced alteration of enzyme levels decreases the effectiveness of the ingested opiates, requiring higher doses to achieve euphoria; but higher doses beget higher tolerance. Meanwhile, the brain perceives that it doesn't need its own endogenous opioids, because heroin is present in abundance. So the endogenous opioids (enkephalin) factory shuts down. Now the brain must rely completely on exogenous substances to relieve anxiety and stress. Remove the drug, and the result is raw panic. Since there's no enkephalin available to regulate the release of GABA (Fig. 3.6), the increased GABA decreases the flow of dopamine into the nucleus accumbens (the Reward Center), resulting in craving and agitation.

The brain, it seems, will not stand for massive chemical overload, and it finds ways to punish those who would tamper with its delicate workings in such a crude way. Most drug users have some intimation of this early in the game: hangovers, crashes, episodes of extreme anxiety and nausea—a vast array of unpleasant warning signals and side effects. Yet the users persist. Why?

It is easier to discuss the chemical process of addiction than its underlying psychological (and possibly physical) causes, but research has given us some insights into the question of why some people seem prone to addiction while others are more resistant, regardless of their behavior. Sadly, the body of evidence suggests that an unhappy few may be biochemically drawn to addiction, like a moth to flame.

Pick Your Parents Carefully

How many times have we heard the following comments?

> I can drink as much as I want and not become an alcoholic.
>
> I can use cocaine recreationally and not become addicted.

On the other hand, we also hear these:

> The only way I can control my drinking is not to drink at all.
>
> After one or two episodes involving cocaine, I was hooked.

All these individuals could be telling the truth. Why? Because different people react differently to the same drug or experience. Clearly, some people seem to be more addiction-prone than others. The Reward Cascade model allows a plausible explanation of this phenomenon. Apparently, for either genetic or environmental reasons, some people have abnormally low neurotransmission in important pathways in the Reward System, including, quite possibly, the nucleus accumbens. This neurotransmitter deficit may manifest itself in feelings of anxiety, craving, and low self-esteem. To alleviate these feelings, the addiction-prone person may resort to drugs that stimulate the flow of neurotransmitters into the reward pathway.

Once the euphoria of the drug has worn off, neurotransmission falls below the predrug level, resulting in even greater anxiety, depression, and craving.

Attempts to regain this euphoria may be the basis for switching stimuli when one particular drug or activity doesn't work anymore. Many people quit one addiction only to become involved in another. These people treat themselves like lab experiments: add a little of this, and if that doesn't work, add a little of something else. A little up, a little down! Or, in the case described in these lines in the song by Travis Tritt and Marty Stuart, substitute a little promiscuous sex for alcohol:

> Women, warm and willing
> Is what I'm looking for
> Because the whiskey
> Ain't doing it, anymore.

One of us once received a letter from a distraught husband who was worried about his wife, a recovering alcoholic, drug addict, and bulimic. She had recently taken up running and other forms of aerobic exercise. She exercised vigorously for more than two hours a day and deeply resented the fact that she did not have time to exercise at least five hours a day. Small amounts of food ingestion would be followed by vigorous exercise to "burn it off." This nearly textbook case of addiction-switching illustrates the hypothesis we proposed many years ago in our book *Craving for Ecstasy:* that activities can become addicting through neurochemical pathways similar to those involved in substance abuse.

Obviously, powerful mind-altering drugs or activities that dramatically overpower synaptic homeostasis are not the answer to the molecular imbalances that may be present in the brains of addiction-prone people. Their health and well-being will be much better served by consistent activities that create a pleasurable but not highly euphoric feeling, activities we will discuss in more detail in later chapters.

But it's important to keep in mind that this admonition is equally true for the individual who is not "addiction-prone." It's all too easy to dismiss all addiction as a product of bad genetic wiring, which implies that the key to optimal living is to "pick your parents carefully." Yet even people who are not prone to addiction can make plenty of unwise choices in their pursuit of pleasure. People who say they can use drugs as much as they want and not become addicts are playing with neurochemical fire. Constantly challenging molecular homeostasis may bring about permanent neurochemical changes virtually indistinguishable from those associated with genetic abnormalities. So, even if you have picked your parents carefully, you should not challenge the brain to a game of molecular roulette. You won't win! After all, we know that certain lifestyles (smoking, overeating, getting no exercise) can induce diseases such as diabetes, obesity, heart trouble, and atherosclerosis. At the very least, alcoholism and other forms of drug addiction should be included in this list, as self-destructive lifestyle choices.

Besides, now you know—because of the brain's tendency to restore synaptic homeostasis, it is neurochemically impossible to maintain a state of exulted euphoria for long periods. As the late Sidney Cohen once wrote, "Brain circuitry permits momentary ecstasy or prolonged pleasure. Apparently, sustained ecstasy is neurophysiologically impossible."

Molecular Madness: Neurotransmission Gone Berserk

Not all problematic chemical imbalances in the brain are self-induced through the use of drugs or participation in compulsive activities. Sometimes the brain seems to lose control of the chemical factory on its own, without any external help. When this occurs, the effects can be devastating.

> A caged bird in spring knows quite well that he might serve some end; he is well aware that there is something for him to do, but he cannot do it. What is it? He does not quite remember. Then some vague ideas occur to him, and he says to himself, "The others build their nests and lay their eggs and bring up their little ones"; and he knocks his head against the bars of the cage. But the cage remains, and the bird is maddened by anguish. "Look at that lazy animal," says another bird in passing, "he seems to be living at ease."
>
> Yes, the prisoner lives, he does not die; there are no outward signs of what passes within him—his health is good, he is more or less gay when the sun shines. But then the season of migration comes, and attacks of melancholia—"But he has everything he wants," say the

children that tend him in his cage. He looks through the bars at the overcast sky where a thunderstorm is gathering, and inwardly he rebels against his fate. "I am caged, I am caged, and you tell me I do not want anything, fools! You think I have everything I need! Oh! I beseech you liberty, that I may be a bird like other birds!"

A certain idle man resembles this idle bird. And circumstances often prevent men from doing things, prisoners in I do not know what horrible, horrible, most horrible cage. There is also—I know it—the deliverance, the tardy deliverance. A justly or unjustly ruined reputation, poverty, unavoidable circumstances, adversity—that is what makes men prisoners.

One cannot always tell what it is that keeps us shut in, confines us, seems to bury us; nevertheless, one feels certain barriers, certain gates, certain walls. Is all this imagination, fantasy? I don't think so. And one asks, "My God! is it for long, is it forever, is it for all eternity?"

These words, written by Vincent van Gogh in July 1880 to his brother, Theo, reflect the internal agony and turmoil that marked most of van Gogh's life. While such utter despair may be reserved for only an unhappy few, many of us have had some intimation of "walls" and "barriers" in our own minds over which we have no control; at one time or another, all of us may have felt, like Baudelaire, "the wind of the wing of madness."

More than a century after van Gogh raged against his plight, we are still puzzling over the causes and treatment of mental illness. Some disorders are so exotic that they have yet to be properly named, let alone understood; yet the form of mental illness that has been studied most extensively happens to be the one that is still the most pervasive: depression. Depression has been dubbed by William Styron as "the gray drizzle of horror." He describes his personal battle with depression in his book *Darkness Visible:*

As the disorder gradually took full possession of my system, I began to conceive that my mind itself was like one of those outmoded smalltown telephone exchanges, being gradually inundated by floodwaters: one by one, the normal circuits began to drown, causing some of the functions of the body and nearly all of those of instinct and intellect to slowly disconnect.

Severe depression robs us of the ability to experience happiness or even a sense of normalcy. Styron continues:

By the time we arrived at the museum, having dealt with heavy traffic, it was past four o'clock and my brain had begun to endure its familiar siege: panic and dislocation, and a sense that my thought processes were being engulfed by a toxic and unnameable tide that obliterated any enjoyable response to the living world.

Too often, victims of this "gray drizzle" can see no escape from their unrelenting agony, and at least 20 percent of depressed people elect suicide as a favorable alternative. Styron describes the agony of their particular form of molecular madness:

The pain of severe depression is quite unimaginable to those who have not suffered it, and it kills in many instances because its anguish can no longer be borne.

Death was now a daily presence, blowing over me in cold gusts. I had not conceived precisely how my end would come. . . . I was still keeping the idea of suicide at bay. But plainly the possibility was around the corner and I would soon meet it face to face.

Many of the artifacts in my house had become potential devices for my own destruction: the attic rafters (and an outside maple or two) a means to hang myself, the garage a place to inhale carbon monoxide, the bathtub a vessel to receive the flow from my opened arteries. The kitchen knives in their drawers had but one purpose for me.

Depression can vary in intensity and length from a few days of the "blahs" to years of nearly nonfunctional existence and excruciating agony. Rod Steiger, who won an Academy award for *In the Heat of the Night,* suffered a depression so severe that for several years he was unable to work:

I had a depression that took me out of the business for almost eight— let's say ten years. A whole generation, who were 25 and now are 35, are in executive positions. I have to remind them that I am alive.

In addition to the living hell that "molecular madness" imposes on its victims, depression and other forms of neurochemical disasters cost the United States more than $100 billion a year in lost production and medical expenses.

What has happened to the ordinarily smooth-functioning, computerlike brain, to produce this kind of suffering? How can the brain, in all its complexity, lose control of its own mood-regulating chemistry? Styron likens the situation to a kind of electronic over-load—an intriguing analogy, and an intuitive one. It it precisely be-cause it is so complex that the brain occasionally loses molecular control—sometimes for short periods, sometimes for months or years or even permanently. The surprise is not that the brain occa-sionally malfunctions but, with its billions of neurons making tril-lions of connections, that it functions so remarkably well.

Although there are many theories regarding the chemical compo-nent of mental illness, virtually all of them focus on a molecular im-balance that brings about a dysregulation of the dynamic and ex-tremely complex mechanisms in the brain. At this point, it should be no surprise to the reader that it is those molecules we call neuro-transmitters which are responsible for this malfunction.

It was originally thought that depression, like other malfunctions of the brain, could be explained as an imbalance of a single neuro-transmitter. For example, depression was once attributed primarily to a deficiency of norepinephrine in certain receptor sites in the brain. Conversely, an excess of norepinephrine was believed to be responsible for the manic phase of bipolar disorder, an affliction in which the sufferer alternates from nearly uncontrolled elation to equally uncontrolled agony.

Neither scenario is now accepted as a complete picture of the problem. Although norepinephrine deficiency appears to be in-volved, the brain is far too complex to permit such a simplistic solu-tion to the wide range of behavioral symptoms grouped under the rather innocuous name depression—a label that trivializes the mag-nitude of the illness. Until we have a better understanding of how the brain operates in the absence of mental illness, we will be unable to comprehend the nature of diseases of the brain.

For the brain to understand itself is, as Colin McGinn has put it, "like monkeys trying to do physics." But like the monkeys, we can at least try. As in the case of the "normal" brain discussed earlier, our description of the processes involved in abnormal neurochemis-try must be somewhat simplistic because of the scope of this book and the limited knowledge currently available. Still, even a cursory discussion of the chemical aspects of mental illness sheds additional light on our theme: the degree to which brain chemistry exerts an inescapable influence over mind, mood, and behavior.

As we noted above, norepinephrine levels appear to play a role in the development of depression. Nevertheless, more recent research by Herbert Meltzer at the Case Western Reserve University School of Medicine suggests an additional powerful role for another neuro-transmitter—you guessed it—serotonin. The evidence that seroto-nin—or, rather, its absence—has something to do with depression is overwhelming. Some of the most convincing evidence comes from studies by P. L. Delgado of the West Haven Veterans Administration Medical Center.

Delgado found that depressed patients who were in remission due to administration of antidepressants suffered reversal of their remis-sion when provided with diets low in tryptophan. Recall that trypto-phan is converted into serotonin in the brain. Not only does trypto-phan depletion have a negative effect on the mood of depressed patients, but Simon Young of McGill University has shown that a diet low in tryptophan brings about a rapid lowering of mood in "normal" subjects.

At the Massachusetts Institute of Technology, Judith and Richard Wurtman have bestowed scientific respectability on Grandmother's milk-and-cookie remedy for sleeplessness (sleep disorder happens to be one of the symptoms of depression). They studied individuals af-flicted with such disorders as carbohydrate craving obesity (CCO), premenstrual syndrome (PMS), and seasonal affective disorder (SAD). They found that the between-meal snacks of CCO and PMS subjects consisted mostly of carbohydrates. They proposed that these individuals snack not because they are hungry, but because carbohydrate-rich foods improve their mood.

When carbohydrate cravers were asked why they succumb to foods they know will exacerbate their obesity, their explanation sounded much like the one provided by SAD sufferers. It almost never had to do with hunger or with the taste of the food; instead, most said they eat to combat tension, anxiety, or mental fatigue. The majority reported that, after eating, they felt calm and clearheaded.

So now we have both serotonin and norepinephrine deficiencies to help explain the wide range of behavioral symptoms common to most depressions. It is possible that a sufficient supply of both neu-rotransmitters may be necessary to alleviate depression. Oren Kalus of the Albert Einstein College of Medicine and others believe that the best treatment for depression is to ensure an adequate concentra-tion of both serotonin and norepinephrine.

Chronic and severe depression is but one example of brain chemistry run amok. Disorders such as schizophrenia, Parkinson's disease, Huntington's chorea and Tourette's syndrome have also been linked to faulty neurochemistry. Such serious illnesses effectively block access to the pathways to pleasure we will be discussing in future chapters and may well require a lifetime of medical care. In time, perhaps, our emerging understanding of brain chemistry may provide better treatment and even relief from these mysterious neuronal torments.

Natural Highs and Prolonged Pleasure

In the absence of debilitating mental illness, most of us have a great deal of choice in how we set about managing our moods, our behavior, and our quest for pleasure. We can seek out intense, mood-altering drugs or activities—a smorgasbord that includes everything from cocaine, alcohol, marijuana, and cigarettes to promiscuous sex, compulsive gambling, and excessive exercise—and run the risk of becoming chemically or psychologically dependent on those drugs or activities for our sense of well-being, to the point of adopting a dysfunctional and addictive lifestyle. Or we can settle for less startling, less dramatic, yet ultimately more sustainable mind-altering experiences, the pathways to pleasure that we have termed natural highs.

The choice is a real one. Brain chemistry makes no fine distinction between jolts of pleasure achieved by artificial means and those which are part of "natural" processes; it's all chemistry. The difference manifests itself only in the long-term effects on the individual. For example, the chemical structure of norepinephrine and amphetamine are nearly identical (Fig. 3.7); both have the ability to elicit a euphoric state.

Yet while one plays a crucial role in the body's defense mechanisms, the other is a dangerous synthetic drug, the ingestion of which results, in many cases, in addiction, declining health, and even death.

The dangers of constantly upsetting synaptic homeostasis in the quest for a bigger and bigger jolt—sustained ecstasy—can best be illustrated by thinking of the brain as a kind of coiled spring. Any spring has a limit of extension, beyond which it should not be

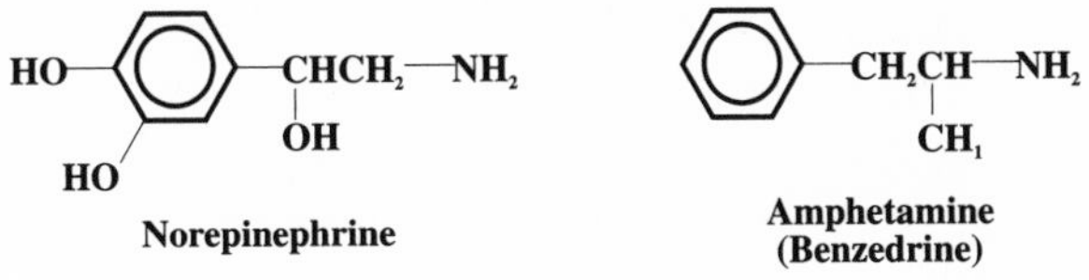

FIGURE 3.7
*Structural Similarity between Norepinephrine
and Amphetamine*

stretched. If one avoids stretching the spring beyond this limit, it can be stretched and relaxed almost indefinitely. This is similar to the stretching of synaptic homeostasis through healthy pleasures, or natural highs. This type of stretching is what the brain is designed to do in order to provide us with the ability to alter our moods, a need all of us have to survive the trials of life. If, however, we insist on stretching the spring beyond the intended limit, we have the potential to severely damage it to the point where it is unable to return to its normal unstretched position. This is analogous to exposure to powerful drugs, which create such an excessive synaptic imbalance that a return to normal predrug neurotransmission may be difficult or even impossible. Thus, the key to optimal living is to select those activities which do not overstretch the synaptic spring, but provide the needed relief from the stress we all encounter. In this instance, *less* may actually mean *more;* in the following chapters, we will address how proper management of nutrition and exercise and the development of a variety of personal coping skills can refine and enhance the experience of healthy pleasures throughout life.

Natural highs, like any skill, must be regularly cultivated and rehearsed. What better way to do this than to never let a day go by without a gentle pull on your synaptic pleasure spring. The key to finding the many pathways to pleasure is to look for them every day, and also not to look so far down the road that one fails to "eat the strawberries along the way." Not a day should pass without consciously seeking out some activity that helps to perk up the neurotransmitters. What can we do to accomplish this? Actually, there is no shortage of neurotransmitter-releasing activities: laugh, sing, run, eat your favorite dessert, cuddle your pet (or child or spouse), make love, play with grandchildren, bicycle, play tennis, work, cry, dance, talk, be silent, meditate, sleep. In other words, live and do it today. The words of the Sanskrit writer express the essence of the pathways to pleasure:

> Look to this day! For it is life, the very life of life, . . . for yesterday is already a dream, and tomorrow is only a vision; but today, well lived, makes every yesterday a dream of happiness, and every tomorrow a vision of hope.

Skill Development

4

Using Your Inner Resources

Here's the thing, say Shug. The thing I believe. God is inside you and inside everybody else. You come into the world with God. But only them that search for it inside find it. And sometimes it just manifest itself even if you not looking, or don't know what you looking for. Though trouble do it for most folks, I think. And sorrow.

It? I asked. Yuh. God ain't a he or a she, but a It.

What do It look like, I asked.

Don't look like nothing, she say. It ain't a picture show. It ain't somethin' you can look at apart from anything else, including yourself. I believe God in everything, say Shug. Everything that is, or ever was, or ever will be. And when you can feel that, and be happy to feel that, you've found It.

—Alice Walker
The Color Purple

This chapter is about developing personal skills for optimal living. While Chapter 2: Nurturing the Healthy Child and Chapter 3: The Chemical Brain provide the mental preparation for natural highs, understanding alone is insufficient for realizing pleasure and meaning throughout the lifespan. Fulfillment is based on the continued satisfaction derived from engaging our creative potential. As stated by Mihaly Csikszentmihalyi in *Flow: The Psychology of Optimal Experience*, "The optimal state of inner experience is one in which there is order in consciousness . . . when psychic energy—or attention—is invested in realistic goals, and when skills match the opportunities for action." People who are invested in forward movement—stretching themselves beyond their existing talents—become extraordinary individuals. They develop a state of "flow," or optimal inner experience, by becoming so involved in an activity that nothing else seems to matter.

Yet the world is rife with tormented geniuses, some of whom have delivered the most complex and beautiful manifestations of human creativity. Abandoning oneself to the pursuit of excellence can itself lead to a distortion of human values and a diminution of pleasure. People become trapped by an ideal of perfection, and their whole life may become centered on exquisite performance. Parents may value their children in accord with how well they can model an idealized vision of what they should be. Performing becomes everything, as natural being is increasingly repressed. This generation has seen the birth of athlete addicts who abuse steroids in pursuit of performance ideals: faster, stronger, higher, farther. The industrialized nations, notably Japan, Germany, and the United States, are engaged in ferocious competition to create the "impeccable product." Preoccupation with excellence occurred in its worst form in Nazi Germany, where people were guided by an ideal of trying to create a race of superhumans. According to Marion Woodman, author of *Addiction to Perfection,* "If you are living for an ideal, and driving yourself as hard as you can to be perfect—at your job or as a mother or as a perfect wife—you lose the natural, slow rhythm of life. There's a rushing, trying to attain the ideal; the slower pace of the beat of the earth, the state where you simply are is forgotten." Ultimately, extended pleasure depends on a continuing sense of purpose—the ability to relate enjoyable activities to goals and values that serve as guiding principles of one's life.

Alice Walker's character Shug points us toward what she perceives as the genuine source of human fulfillment—finding a unity between all things. "I believe God in everything, say Shug. . . . And when you can feel that, and be happy to feel that, you've found It." A fundamental premise of this book is that optimal living depends on the attainment of peace of mind—a sense of inner harmony—often linked to spiritual growth and development. When a person can combine the experience of *integration,* knowing how he or she fits in the scheme of all things, with *differentiation,* the unique expression of increasingly complex skills and talents, natural highs are the inevitable result.

In this chapter, we begin by exploring plausible means of feeling integrated, or relaxed, in this awesome and turbulent world. Many have found peace of mind through making contact with an energy that to them represents the unity and purpose of all things: God. It is becoming recognized in psychological circles that somehow the spirit must be attended to, as well as the mind. Some refer to the spiritual part of us that needs nurturing and attention as the "creative self," the part of us that discovers or uncovers beauty and harmony.

Psychotherapist Thomas Moore simply refers to it as the soul, and in his well-regarded book *Care of the Soul* he defines it this way: "Let us imagine the care of the soul, then as the application of poetics in everyday life . . . [C]are of the soul is a fundamentally different way of regarding daily life and the quest for happiness. The emphasis may not be on problems at all. One person might care for the soul by buying or renting a good piece of land, another by painting his house or his bedroom. Care of the soul is a continuous process that concerns itself not so much with fixing a central flaw as with attending to the small details of everyday life."

Spiritual Quests

To find God, the things that people do—aside from prayer—include eating and not eating, asceticism and self-flagellation, sitting, dancing, singing, chanting, reciting hymns, painting, taking drugs, observing everything, observing nothing, focusing on a single thought or sensation (e.g., the very act of breathing), communing with others, seeking solitary quietude, and, more recently, plugging themselves into a personalized mind machine—a device that uses special frequency lights and sounds to alter their brain waves. Why all this fuss?

As Aldous Huxley observed, we seek access to the spiritual world in the belief that it is more beautiful and real than the actual world in which we live. We struggle with how to let go of youth, vigor, and the people we love, and with how to quiet the mind's nervous chatter about deterioration, death, or fear of nonbeing. Indeed, there is a universal quest to catch but a glimpse of perfection and harmony—eternal beauty and continuous ecstasy. Margaret Prescott Montague writes:

My eyes were opened, and for the first time in all my life I caught a glimpse of the ecstatic beauty of reality. It was not an experience for words. It was an emotion. A rapture of the heart. I knew that every man, woman, bird and tree, every living thing before me, was extravagantly beautiful and extravagantly important. I saw no new thing, but I saw all the usual things in a new, miraculous light, in what I believe was their true light. I saw for the first time how wildly beautiful and joyous, beyond any words of mine to describe, is the whole of life. For those fleeting moments I did indeed love my neighbor as myself.

Transcendence is so highly prized that throughout the ages, people have taken extraordinary measures—psychological, physiological, and chemical—to induce visions of spirituality or splendor. Here we review varied practices for gaining access to the spiritual domain. Yet this section should be regarded not as a pathway to heaven but, rather, as an exploration of means to achieve peace of mind, the mental substrate for natural highs.

One method of altering perception is sensory isolation. This may be achieved by seeking out or creating environments where ordinary sensations such as light, sound, temperature, and even gravity are minimized or, in some cases, eliminated almost entirely. John Lilly, author of *Center of the Cyclone,* devised a means for reducing external stimuli so that the information he received from the outside world was practically nil. In essence, he immersed himself in a bath of salt water that was kept at body temperature, breathed through a snorkel so that his face was completely covered (thus, no part of his skin was feeling anything but a uniform temperature), and tied himself up in a harness that didn't permit him to move more than a tenth of an inch—all of this in a light- and sound-proof environment. Within four hours, Lilly and those who modeled his experiment were able to induce strange visions, some of which were thought of as transcendent.

Lilly's experiments, which spawned a generation of "float to relax" tanks, are miniversions of isolation practices that have been carried on through the ages. Prophets typically found themselves— by either choice or circumstance—in the most desolate habitats on earth. In fourth-century Egypt, for example, a large number of religious seekers lived in the desert, cutting themselves off from ordinary stimuli. The same practice is observed in Tibetan lamas and Hindu monks who seek out remote caves in the Himalayas.

An interesting cross-cultural similarity is that many visionary incidents are reported to be painful or disagreeable. For example, in museums throughout the world, the Temptation of St. Anthony is almost universally rendered as diabolic visions. Whether they occur in natural desolation or controlled laboratory settings, and whether beatific or dreadful, visionary experiences are nearly always astoundingly intense.

Humankind has managed to forge yet another wedge into the spiritual domain by producing certain alterations in body chemistry. One means to alter our physiological balance is to introduce variation into the normal process of breathing. Practiced for thousands of years in the Orient, prolonged suspensions of breath—sometimes for a minute or even longer—result in an increased amount of carbon dioxide in the blood. It is known that an increase in CO_2, induced either by breathing or by direct inhalation of the gas itself, will produce strange psychological experiences, often regarded as transcendent or unreal. Numerous Eastern views, including Yoga, describe the breath as a spiritual life force (*chi, prana*), an element that cannot be measured but whose power is legend. Devotees believe that when *prana* is increased by special breathing methods and diet, changes in consciousness and increased levels of spirituality ensue.

Like so many well-developed skills and practices, the time-honored Yogic breathing methods also appear in caricature form. Just as subway graffiti can be regarded as an undisciplined form of artistic activity, novices worldwide stumble on means to alter the CO_2 level in their body and brain, leading to extraordinary perceptual experiences. Hyperventilation—rapid breathing—alters perception in relation to reduced levels of brain CO_2. When CO_2 levels drop, the balance of brain acidity shifts, which may also contribute to unusual mental effects. A college professor, now in his midforties, explains how he gained access to strange perceptions through a street ritual that seemed to spontaneously emerge in a lower-middle-class neighborhood of the Bronx. He later learned, through extensive traveling, that what he thought to be unique to his cultural subgroup was practiced by youth around the globe.

One day, when I was about twelve years old, we had just finished a game of stickball and were standing around wondering what to do next. A thirteen-year-old kid from around the block joined the crowd and said he had something new for us to try. I volunteered, thinking that a novel experience was at hand.

The neighborhood guru instructed me to hyperventilate, which he modeled by taking a series of very rapid and shallow breaths. I was then told to coordinate this special breathing technique with ten quickly executed deep-knee-bends. Just as I finished this respiratory exertion, the guru signaled his twelve-year-old sidekick—who seemed to act as a sort of emergency medical technician—to grab me from behind, forcibly depressing the solar plexus, a spot he designated between my ribs and stomach.

I can still vividly remember the eerie feeling of "coming to" in the middle of the gutter; swinging my fists like a boxer in slow motion; regaining consciousness with an awareness of having returned from a cosmic darkness, brushed with an essence that reminded me of war, heroism, and death.

It was such an interesting experience that I repeated it again and again.

On hearing this account, somewhere between 10 and 20 percent of our audiences from many places in the world—Brazil, Iceland, Turkey, Australia—report a similar discovery during childhood. In almost every case, the experience seemed so weird or idiosyncratic to their neighborhood or clique that they never told anyone about it. Many people, particularly students who are now in their early twenties, report that they came on an even quicker method to achieve the same state: simply grab your friend around the neck, cutting off blood to the carotid artery (one of two main vessels carrying blood to the head), causing the person to faint almost immediately.

Another method to create unusual perceptual experiences is through fasting. Indians in the United States and other areas of the world have habitually and systematically used fasting as an initiation rite for the express purpose of achieving visionary experiences. To a considerable extent, fasting is also used in all the world religions. In Judaism, for example, Yom Kippur—the Day of Atonement, the most solemn day of the Jewish year—is observed with a fast that extends from dusk to dusk. The ensuing feast is punctuated with hearty appropriations of wine. During Ramadan, the ninth month of the Moslem year, rigid fasting is observed during all daylight hours.

Similarly, going without or cutting down on sleep will also cause dramatic psychological effects. Also, some of the more violent physical austerities, such as self-flagellation, undoubtedly produce chemical changes that facilitate transcendent experiences. The ritual practice of inserting hooks in one's body and spears through the cheeks or tongue is annually celebrated by Hindu devotees in Malaysia. Augmented by frenetic music, chanting, intense heat, incense, and colorful representations of Hindu deities carried on their backs, pilgrims release great quantities of histamine, endorphin, and adrenalin, the combined effect of which may have profound psychological effects.

Beyond these behavioral methods of inducing religious experiences, there are the directly chemical techniques. In one of a series of lectures on "What a Piece of Work Is Man," Aldous Huxley addressed the phenomenon of chemically induced visionary experiences:

> A really startling fact about recent pharmacological developments is that a number of chemical substances have been produced, discovered in recent years, which permit the opening of the door into the visionary world without inflicting serious damage upon the body. . . . [A friend] told me that he recently returned from Mexico and had gone down there to visit an old witch doctor, his friend there, bringing her a number of the pills [LSD] which Hofmann had synthesized, which she had taken and was quite delighted because they produced exactly the same effect as the mushrooms, and she was especially delighted because now she could practice her magic every season of the year instead of having to wait for the mushroom season! So this is one of the great triumphs of modern science, that the witch doctor will be able to send a postcard to Dr. Hofmann in Basel saying, "Have important magic to do. Please send 100 capsules air mail."

Huxley was obviously enchanted with the possibility of discovering a pathway to enlightenment in a pill. In the *Doors of Perception,* his eloquent description of twelve hours under the influence of a single capsule of mescaline, he commented:

> To others again is revealed the glory, the infinite value and meaningfulness of naked existence, of the given, unconceptualized event. In

the final stage of egolessness there is an obscure knowledge that All is in awe—that Awe is actually each. This is as near, I take it, as a finite mind can ever come to perceiving anything that is happening everywhere in the universe.

Of course, loss of one's sense of self—ego dissolution, in the jargon of modern psychiatry—is risky business. At one point during his psychedelic journey, Huxley felt himself on the brink of panic:

This, I suddenly thought, was going too far. Too far, even though the going was into intenser beauty, deeper significance. The fear as I analyzed it in retrospect, was of being overwhelmed, of disintegrating under a pressure of reality greater than a mind, accustomed to living most of the time in a cozy world of symbols, could possibly bear.

For decades, movie audiences have been given a filmmaker's version of the chemical experience. From *Easy Rider* to *Woodstock* to *The Doors*, movies have tried to re-create the colorful and spontaneous disassociation from mundane reality that a good drug experience is supposed to provide. Even relatively innocent films like Disney's *Fantasia* and Kubrick's *2001: A Space Odyssey* were rumored to contain passages directly inspired by drug use, and said to be visually accurate depictions of an LSD trip or an opium dream.

According to Soloman Snyder, director of the Department of Neuroscience at Johns Hopkins University, the panic precipitated by psychedelics can be cataclysmic. Intense fear merging with terror and disorientation have caused many people to commit suicide. Others have become psychotic under the drug's influence and failed to emerge after dissipation of the drug's pharmacological effects. According to Snyder, "hundreds of cases of schizophrenic illness have been precipitated by a single psychedelic experience. The possibility that they may initiate a long term mental illness is perhaps the most serious danger presented by psychedelic drugs."

Peaceful Body, Peace of Mind

Profoundly different—even mystical and sometimes terrorizing—experiences can arise from an array of mind-altering techniques. But the spiritual quest is often motivated by a fundamental wish to find peace through connecting with the oneness and ultimate harmony of all things. Walt Whitman writes:

Swiftly arose and spread around me the peace and joy and knowledge that passes all the art and argument of the earth; and I know that the hand of God is the elder hand of my own and I know that the Spirit of God is the eldest brother of my own.

As we have shown through repeated examples in Chapter 3: The Chemical Brain, the more invasive modifiers of conscious experience exact a precious toll by causing the body to defend against neuro-chemical maelstroms. Baba Ram Dass, alias Richard Alpert, Ph.D., experimented with various psychedelics. At one point, he and five others locked themselves in a building for three weeks and took 400 micrograms of LSD every four hours. In *Be Here Now,* he describes his disillusionment and final abandonment of what he thought was a spiritual journey:

> For five years I dealt with the matter of "coming down." The coming down matter is what led me to the next chapter of this drama. Because after six years I realized that no matter how ingenious my experimental designs were, and how high I got, I came down.
> . . . We finally were just drinking out of the bottle, because it didn't seem to matter anymore. We'd just stay at a plateau, we were very high. What happened in those three weeks in that house, no one would ever believe, including us. At the end of those three weeks, we walked out of the house and within a few days, we came down!
> And it was a terribly frustrating experience. As if you came into the kingdom of heaven and you saw how it all was and you felt these new states of awareness, and then you got cast out again, and after two or three hundred times of this, began to feel an extraordinary kind of depression set in—a very gentle depression that whatever I knew still wasn't enough!

Peace of mind must be approached through gentler means, such as the meditative and relaxation practices that occupy a vital place in Eastern and Western psychology.

But how should one select from the panoply of practices, all touted as effective combatants in the omnipresent struggle to conquer stress? First, we acknowledge that two general types of anxiety exist: mental and physical. Consider, for example, a person who lies down, eyes wide open, unable to sleep because her mind is "racing out of control." While this woman is experiencing *cognitive* anxiety, her spouse, lying only six inches away, begins to toss and turn. As his stomach feels tense, his muscles can't seem to relax. He is experiencing *somatic* anxiety.

Given that these two broad problems exist, readers may develop a relaxation practice that is compatible with their style of responding to stress. Table 4.1 summarizes some common self-soothing techniques. Although a thorough review is beyond the scope of this chapter, the section on references and notes provides additional resources.

In *The Meditative Mind,* Daniel Goleman, behavioral science reporter for the *New York Times,* provides an overview of Eastern spiritual pathways that have evolved during the past 4,000 years. He wrote the first part of his book while living in a tiny Himalayan village during the monsoon season in 1971. At this time, meditation was unfamiliar to the Western psyche. Goleman felt he needed a Baedeker, "a traveler's guide to this topography of the spirit." Now, after more than two decades, things have changed significantly. It is common for Westerners today to admit they view meditation as potentially beneficial to their lives, and millions have incorporated Eastern teaching into their schedules. Meditation is now accepted practice in all healing and human services professions: medicine, psychology and education, to name but a few.

Goleman's research on Eastern spiritual thought involved several months of study with Indian yogis and swamis, Tibetan lamas, and southern Buddhist laymen and monks: "Strange terms and concepts assailed me: 'samadhi,' 'jhana,' 'turiya,' 'nirvana,' and a host of others used by these teachers to explain their spiritual paths. Each path seemed to be in essence the same as every other path, but each had his own way of travelling it and what major landmarks to expect." Goleman felt confused about how to organize the diverse spiritual knowledge he had recently acquired. Just then, Joseph Goldstein, a Buddhist meditation teacher, triggered a flash of insight: "It's simple mathematics. All meditation systems either aim for One or Zero—union with God or emptiness. The path to the One is through concentration on Him, to the Zero is insight into the voidness of one's mind."

Before learning the fundamentals of these prototypical relaxation techniques, readers are invited to consider how the antithesis of calm—stress—figures into their quest for optimal living. Meditation will then be more clearly understood as an invaluable skill whenever life takes the inevitable turn of intense change.

The Stress Factor

Psychologists have long known that people perform most effectively when under some degree of stress. A moderate level of arousal tends to produce alertness and enthusiasm for the task at hand. When emotional excitement exceeds an optimal level, however, whether the evoked feelings are positive or negative, the result is progressive impairment of one's ability to function. Not only do stress victims show signs of diminished mental capacity, but their physical health begins to deteriorate as well. Nearly forty years ago, Hans Selye, the grandfather of stress research, found illness and death to be the inevitable result of prolonged stress.

When we become excited, through either anger or fear, the brain signals hormone-producing glands to prepare us for fight or flight. The adrenal glands produce cortisol, a chemical that increases blood sugar and speeds up the body's metabolism. Other messages to the adrenal glands result in the release of the amphetaminelike stimulant epinephrine (adrenaline), which helps supply glucose to the muscles and brain, and norepinephrine, which speeds up the heart rate and elevates blood pressure.

The psychological byproducts of a moderate biochemical emergency are noticeable increments in one's feelings of physical prowess and personal competence, often associated with strong sensations of pleasure. In many ways, the state of biological and psychological "readiness" produced by stress is mimicked by the effects of stimulant drugs. People may self-induce similar alterations of consciousness with amphetamines, cocaine, or caffeine (two and a half cups of coffee will double the level of epinephrine in the blood), or by engaging in activities that appear to be life-threatening. Positive experiences—falling in love, riding a roller coaster, watching a great theatrical performance—can evoke the same stress hormones as more troublesome flirtations with danger or drugs. Selye has been acutely aware of the intoxicating correlates of flight-or-fight reactions. He points to stress drunkenness as causing more overall harm to society than the universally acclaimed demon of demons, alcohol. One can-

TABLE 4.1

Common Self-Soothing Techniques

Progressive Relaxation	Hypnotic Suggestion	Autogenic Training
The most extensive relaxation technique used today. The effectiveness of brief training is well established. This method involves the systematic focus of attention on the various gross-muscle groups throughout the body. Subjects are first instructed to actively tense each group for a few seconds after which they are told to release the muscles and relax, e.g., "When I say 'Let go,' I want you to stop tensing, immediately, and simply concentrate on what these muscles feel like as you learn to relax."	Hypnotic suggestions of relaxation typically involve generating soothing thoughts or images; e.g., subjects may be asked to imagine a peaceful day at the beach, with waves gently rolling on the sand.	The core of this procedure is passive attention to bodily processes. Autogenic training typically involves the subject leaning back in an armchair with her or his eyes closed in a quiet room. Verbal formulas are introduced, and the subject is instructed to "passively concentrate" on repetition.
The sequence of tension, release, and attention is sequentially applied to the following muscle groups: dominant hand and forearm; dominant upper arm, nondominant hand and forearm, forehead,	Successful completion of a hypnotic suggestion usually involves a shift in one's focus of thought from the external environment to internally generated mental activity. An important component in the execution of a hypnotist's suggestion is the active generation of imagery with occasional attention to bodily processes, e.g., "Imagine you are holding something heavy in your hand. . . . Now the hand and arm feel heavy, as if the weight were pressing down."	The formulas consist of verbal suggestions intended to facilitate concentration and "mental contact" with specific parts of the body, e.g., the right arm. Training usually begins with the theme of heaviness, and the first formula is "My right arm is heavy." Heaviness training is then continued for each extremity.

eyes and nose, cheeks and mouth, neck and throat, chest, back, and respiratory muscles, abdomen, dominant upper leg and calf, foot, nondominant upper leg, calf and foot. Progression to each muscle group is dependent on complete relaxation of the prior group.

The major emphasis of this method is on *somatic* relaxation.

These techniques that offer active cognitive self-regulation may be more effective for people who have the ability to produce vivid mental images.

The major emphasis of this method is on *cognitive* relaxation.

The next group of formulas involve warmth and begins with "My right arm is warm." Following warmth training in all the limbs, there is usually passive concentration on cardiac activity through the formula "Heartbeat calm and regular." Focus then shifts to the respiratory system via "It breathes me," and warmth in the abdominal region. "My solar plexus is warm." Finally, the last formula is introduced, "My forehead is cool."

Like progressive relaxation, the primary emphasis of autogenic training is on somatic relaxation.

Source: Adapted from Davidson, R.J. and Schwartz, G. E. The Psychobiology of relaxation and related states: a multi-process theory. In D. I. Mostofsky (Ed.) *Behavior Control and Modification of Physiological Processes.* New York: Prentice-Hall, 1976.

not help but wonder if the operative factor behind many of our fallen icons (e.g., Jimmy Swaggart, Gary Hart, and Elvis Presley) is inebriation due to stress.

How, though, does stress actually inflict harm to the body? In sounding the alarm for fight or flight, not only do heart rate, blood sugar, and adrenal activity increase, but a corresponding elevation of fats and cholesterol occurs. The stomach secretes more acid, and the body's immune system slows down. These potentially harmful sequelae are exaggerated as the stresses we face become more numerous, persistent, and severe. Over time, the body may react with such telltale signs as gastrointestinal stress, high blood cholesterol, insomnia, or lower back pain. Most significant, however, is an increased vulnerability to disease. Depending on one's biological makeup, exposure, and life circumstance, stress victims may develop a broad spectrum of life-threatening illnesses, including heart disease, ulcers, and depression, to name just a few.

After Selye's description of the drastic effects of prolonged stress in animals, researchers from the early 1950s to the middle 1970s explored the notion that chronic stress inevitably leads to human illness and death. Typically, hospitalized patients were found to be under more stress prior to their hospitalization than a comparable group of patients who were less ill. In other studies, healthy people filled out a stress questionnaire to measure stress in the preceding six months, after which the researchers waited to see if the high-stress people got sick. Sure enough, those who scored in the upper third of the stress scale had nearly 90 percent more illness in the follow-up period than those who scored in the lower third. In the 1960s, medical researchers Thomas Holmes and Richard Rahe—using a scale score of 100 to denote maximum stress and defining marriage as representing a stress level of 50—developed a checklist of stressful events. The researchers posited that *any* major change, negative or positive, could be stressful; that is, that stress might be incurred equally by such seemingly disparate events as the loss of a loved one and the birth of a long-awaited, healthy baby.

The Holmes-Rahe Scale of Stresses, similar to the one shown in Table 4.2, has been used in literally hundreds of studies. By the mid-1970s, millions of people believed that their level of stress was a strong predictor of whether or not they would become ill. Readers

TABLE 4.2

Scale of Stresses

This is a list of events that occur commonly in people's lives. The numbers in the column headed "Mean Value" indicate how stressful each event is. More specifically, a high number means the event is intensely stressful and will take a long time to adjust to. Thinking about the last year, note the events that happened to you. By each event, indicate the number of times that it occurred in the past twelve months. Multiply this number, or frequency, by the number in the "Mean Value" column. Adding all of these products (event frequency × value) will give you your total stress score for the year. A total score of 150–99 indicates mild life crisis; 200–299, moderate life crisis; and 300+, major life crisis.

Life Event	Mean Value	Stress Index
Death of spouse	_____ × 100 =	_____
Divorce	_____ × 73 =	_____
Marital separation	_____ × 65 =	_____
Jail term	_____ × 63 =	_____
Death of close family member	_____ × 63 =	_____
Personal injury or illness	_____ × 53 =	_____
Marriage	_____ × 50 =	_____
Fired at work	_____ × 47 =	_____
Marital reconciliation	_____ × 45 =	_____
Retirement	_____ × 45 =	_____
Change in health of family member	_____ × 44 =	_____
Pregnancy	_____ × 40 =	_____
Sex difficulties	_____ × 39 =	_____
Gain of new family member	_____ × 39 =	_____
Business readjustment	_____ × 38 =	_____
Change in financial state	_____ × 37 =	_____
Death of close friend	_____ × 36 =	_____
Change to different line of work	_____ × 35 =	_____
Change in number of arguments with spouse	_____ × 31 =	_____
Mortgage more than $10,000	_____ × 30 =	_____
Foreclosure of mortgage or loan	_____ × 29 =	_____
Change in responsibilities at work	_____ × 29 =	_____
Son or daughter leaving home	_____ × 29 =	_____
Trouble with in-laws	_____ × 28 =	_____
Outstanding personal achievement	_____ × 26 =	_____
Spouse beginning or stopping work	_____ × 26 =	_____
Begin or end school	_____ × 25 =	_____
Change in living conditions	_____ × 24 =	_____

TABLE 4.2

(continued)

Life Event	Mean Value	Stress Index
Revision of personal habits	_____ × 23 =	_____
Trouble with boss	_____ × 20 =	_____
Change in work hours or conditions	_____ × 20 =	_____
Change in residence	_____ × 20 =	_____
Change in schools	_____ × 19 =	_____
Change in recreation	_____ × 19 =	_____
Change in church activities	_____ × 18 =	_____
Change in social activities	_____ × 17 =	_____
Mortgage or loan less than $10,000	_____ × 16 =	_____
Change in sleeping habits	_____ × 15 =	_____
Change in number of family get-togethers	_____ × 15 =	_____
Vacation	_____ × 13 =	_____
Christmas	_____ × 12 =	_____
Minor violations of the law	_____ × 11 =	_____

Total = _____

are invited to complete the scale to determine the intensity of their life changes—wanted or unwanted—in the past year.

Yet it is impossible to "Just Say No" to stress. Life imposes constant change, with or without our consent. Further, certain stressful events are opportunities for growth and fulfillment: studying at a university, taking a new job, being pregnant, writing a book, building a home. Would we really enjoy improved health and increased longevity by avoiding the milestones of personal development?

The Metropolitan Life Insurance Company has more than an academic interest in this question. Could insurance premiums be indicated by environmental stressors? In 1974, the company examined 1,078 men who held one of the top three executive jobs in Fortune 500 companies. Metropolitan found a *37 percent lower* mortality rate among these executives than in other males of similar age and cultural background. In 1979, the company conducted another study, this time investigating the mortality rate of 2,352 women listed in *Who's Who*. Their annual deathrate was found to be *25 percent lower* than that of their contemporaries, with the highest rate of heart disease among women in jobs with little security, status, or control. Isn't it likely that successful male executives and renowned female professionals would face high levels of family- and job-related stress by virtue of their stature and achievement orientation? Why, then, do they appear to have a *lower* mortality rate than a more "laid-back" comparison group?

In 1975, Suzanne Kobasa, then a psychology graduate student—who, incidentally, scored very high on the Holmes-Rahe scale—began to research these questions. Intuitively, she did not believe she was a more vulnerable person because of the intense changes in her life. She seized on a once-in-a-lifetime opportunity to study stress: the dissolution of the Bell Telephone Company. It was known that the vast majority of the 700 mid- and upper-level telephone executives she interviewed would lose their jobs as AT&T and Illinois Bell moved into some of the biggest changes in their hundred-year history. These executives' life experiences on the Holmes-Rahe scale would seem to put them at a high risk for illness. Supported by Dr. Robert Hilker, the medical director of Illinois Bell, Kobasa followed these executives over the next eight years, while observing their home and work pressures and the divestiture of AT&T. Nearly all 700 executives filled out two questionnaires: a version of the Holmes-Rahe scale and a checklist of symptoms and illnesses. The 200 executives who scored highest on the Holmes-Rahe scale were then divided into two groups: 100 who stayed healthy, versus 100 who got sick.

Using computer analysis, Kobasa and her colleagues tried to ascertain how to account for health differences between these similarly stressed-out groups. After determining that well-being was unrelated to age, wealth, job status, or education, the researchers wondered whether there might be significant personality differences between the two groups. Perhaps some people resist stress by not becoming aroused in the first place. In other words, if change were not perceived as dangerous—rather, as a life event to be met with confidence—then the toxic results of secreting adrenaline and having compromised immune functions might never become an issue.

Kobasa identified three major personality traits that serve as resiliency factors against stress: (1) commitment—to self, work, family, and other important values; (2) control—a sense of personal control over one's life; and (3) challenge—the ability to see change in one's life as a challenge to master. According to Kobasa, "The stressed but healthy executives were more committed, felt more in control and had bigger appetites for challenge. . . . [O]n some indicators, the healthy executives showed twice as much hardiness. These personality traits were their most potent protection against stress." Readers are now invited to complete The Hardiness Inventory (Table 4.3).

Kobasa and her colleagues reached some rather startling conclusions:

- A hardy personality is more important than a strong constitution.
- Hardy people from sickly families do better under stress than those from healthy families but with fewer inner resources.
- Those who are hardy personalities and exercisers are healthier than those who are only one or the other.
- Hardy people handle conflict better.
- Hardy people can accept "problem focused support" from their families and co-workers and use the support well.
- Hardiness can diffuse Type A personality traits, i.e., lower the risk of coronary heart disease.

Kobasa and other stress management experts believe that hardiness can be developed. Through self-reflection and teaching, one can become more committed, in control, and open to challenge. As shown in Table 4.4, three pathways to hardiness have been described. In view of the inevitability of life stress, learning to improve one's coping skills is certainly worth a try.

Playing to Your Strengths: Defining Your Intellectual Posture

Harvard psychologist Howard Gardner has abandoned the notion that there isn't just one kind of intelligence, but several "frames of mind." As shown in Chapter 1 (Table 1.1), Gardner has specified "Seven Way to Be Bright." His view of intelligence is rooted in biology, and he cites research that convincingly points to different brain regions as the locus of different intellectual and creative abilities. The domains of intelligence Gardner has identified include not only the revered skills of academia—language and mathematics—but also musical skills, spatial skills (the visual skills exhibited by a painter or architect), body-kinesthetic qualities (flexibility and

TABLE 4.3

The Hardiness Inventory

Write down how much you agree or disagree with the following statements, using this scale:

0 = strongly disagree
1 = mildly disagree
2 = mildly agree
3 = strongly agree

_____ A. Trying my best at work makes a difference.
_____ B. Trusting to fate is sometimes all I can do in a relationship
_____ C. I often wake up eager to start on the day's projects.
_____ D. Thinking of myself as a free person leads to great frustration and difficulty.
_____ E. I would be willing to sacrifice financial security in my work if something really challenging came along.
_____ F. It bothers me when I have to deviate from the routine or schedule I've set for myself.
_____ G. An average citizen can have an impact on politics.
_____ H. Without the right breaks, it is hard to be successful in my field.
_____ I. I know why I am doing what I'm doing at my work.
_____ J. Getting close to people puts me at risk of being obligated to them.
_____ K. Encountering new situations is an important priority in my life.
_____ L. I really don't mind when I have nothing to do.

To score yourself: These questions measure control, commitment, and challenge. For half the questions, a high score (like 3, "strongly agree") indicates hardiness; for the other half, a low score (disagreement) does. To figure your scores on control, commitment, and challenge, first enter the number of your answer—0, 1, 2, or 3—in the blank next to the letter of each question on the score sheet. Then add and subtract as shown. (To get your score on "control," add your answers to questions A and G; add your answers to B and H; and then subtract the second number from the first.) Add your scores on commitment, control, and challenge together to get a score for total hardiness. A total score of **10–18** shows a hardy personality; **0–9,** moderate hardiness; and **below 0,** low hardiness.

```
____ + ____ = ____          ____ + ____ = ____          ____ + ____ = ____
 A      G                     C      I                     E      K
              −                                                        −
____ + ____ = ____          ____ + ____ = ____          ____ + ____ = ____
 B      H   Control          D      J  Commitment        F      L  Challenge
       +              +                   =
____        _____        _____        _____
Control   Commitment      Challenge      Total Hardiness Score
```

Source: reprinted with permission of S. Kobasa.

TABLE 4.4
Pathways to Hardiness

Focusing	Restructuring	Self-Improvement
Concentrate on the tension in your body and determine where things are not right, e.g., neck tightness, stomach knots.	Recall a recent episode of stress; then describe how it could have gone better and how it could have gone worse.	Take on a new challenge. Take on a new task, like learning a sport, becoming active in a political or social cause, or embarking on a course of study.
Ask the question, "What factors are preventing me from being at my best today?"	What might someone who handles stress better than you have done?	Self-improvement can reassure you that you can still cope.
Treat yourself kindly; don't punish yourself for poor preparation or performance. Be proud of what you *have* accomplished.	Appreciate that things might have gone more badly.	After the stress is over, avoid self-criticism and take pleasure that the episode has passed.
	When anticipating a future stressor, visualize what may take place. Rehearsal will make the actual event seem more familiar and will enable you to relax and handle the situation more comfortably.	

poise—actions that involve physical skill and coordination), and two "personal intelligences" that involve a graceful understanding of oneself and others.

Among the main implications of Gardner's work is that *applied intelligence*—playing to one's innate intellectual strengths—is a smart way of reducing stress, making maximum use of one's inner resources. According to Gardner, "The gifted adult is that individual who retains much of the spirit and flexibility of the young child, but has wedded it to high levels of achievement within a domain or set of domains." Frank Rainey, consultant to the Colorado Department of Education, has designed means to identify the channels of learning and self-expression that appear to reflect our domains of intelligence. By completing the Multiple Intelligences Profile Indicator (Table 4.5), you can identify the particular "frames of mind" that might be considered your "strong suits" for understanding the uni-

TABLE 4.5
Multiple Intelligences Profile Indicator

Please indicate for the following items the degree to which you think the stated characteristic or behavior fits the individual in question. Circle the appropriate number.

0 = Unsure   1 = Fits not at all   2 = Fits slightly
3 = Fits moderately   4 = Fits strongly

This individual:

1.	Likes to identify or create categories and to sort objects or ideas into categories.	0 1 2 3 4
2.	Is physically very active but generally in very purposeful ways.	0 1 2 3 4
3.	Draws a lot; uses diagrams, sketches, or pictures to help explain or understand ideas and feelings.	0 1 2 3 4
4.	Able to express accurately his/her inner feelings or self-knowledge in a variety of ways.	0 1 2 3 4
5.	Learns to put together complex sequences of physical activities or routines with relative ease.	0 1 2 3 4
6.	Able to follow complex lines of reasoning.	0 1 2 3 4
7.	Likes to read, write or talk a lot.	0 1 2 3 4
8.	Acts on the basis of knowledge of self.	0 1 2 3 4
9.	Likes to act out things, to show physically how something works or can be done.	0 1 2 3 4
10.	Can figure out how to do fairly complex things just by observing the process or looking at pictures or diagrams.	0 1 2 3 4
11.	Very sensitive to the meanings of words and tends to choose words for their exactness or precision.	0 1 2 3 4
12.	Seeks interaction with others; enjoys the challenge of interacting with others.	0 1 2 3 4
13.	Easily creates mental images of things and ideas; is able easily to change or modify mental images of things.	0 1 2 3 4
14.	Very sensitive to rhythm, pitch and qualities of tone in music.	0 1 2 3 4
15.	Likes to build things, take things apart, put things together; may take something apart and put it together again so it is different from the way it was originally.	0 1 2 3 4
16.	Very sensitive to the effect words have on himself/herself or others when reading, writing or speaking.	0 1 2 3 4
17.	Likes to discuss or argue ideas; enjoys finding holes or filling gaps in logical reasoning.	0 1 2 3 4

TABLE 4.5

(continued)

---

18. Understands his/her own inner feelings, motivations and intentions.   0 1 2 3 4
19. Gets along well with others; is likeable and sociable.   0 1 2 3 4
20. Likes to listen to music or to perform music.   0 1 2 3 4
21. Recognizes patterns and relationships among objects and ideas.   0 1 2 3 4
22. Likes to experiment with things in controlled, orderly ways.   0 1 2 3 4
23. Very sensitive to the effect music has on himself/herself or on others.   0 1 2 3 4
24. Able to figure out the way something is done or works or how something is constructed simply by studying the finished product.   0 1 2 3 4
25. Can use his/her hands and fingers with great skill and control.   0 1 2 3 4
26. Likes puns, word games and other humor with words and language.   0 1 2 3 4
27. Economical in the use of body movements.   0 1 2 3 4
28. Very sensitive to the feelings and moods of others.   0 1 2 3 4
29. Individualistic; not unduly concerned about what others might think about him/her.   0 1 2 3 4
30. Often able to figure out the motivations and intentions of others; able to act using knowledge of others.   0 1 2 3 4
31. Has a large vocabulary; likes to use or experiment with new or sophisticated words.   0 1 2 3 4
32. Independent and generally self-assured.   0 1 2 3 4
33. Likes to make up tunes or melodies.   0 1 2 3 4
34. Senses musical elements (rhythm, pitch and qualities of tone) in situations not generally associated with music.   0 1 2 3 4
35. Able to influence others; persuasive.   0 1 2 3 4
36. Has a good sense of timing in physical activities.   0 1 2 3 4
37. Has a strong and accurate inner sense of what he or she wants or needs.   0 1 2 3 4
38. Reads body language well.   0 1 2 3 4
39. Able to devise orderly systems or plans for accomplishing complex tasks.   0 1 2 3 4
40. Likes to improvise with music.   0 1 2 3 4
41. Uses language skillfully to explain things or to show how conclusions have been drawn.   0 1 2 3 4
42. Has a strong sense of composition in art, photography, or interior decorating.   0 1 2 3 4

TABLE 4.5

(continued)

DIRECTIONS FOR SCORING

1. If you circled: 0, score 0
   1, score 0
   2, score 2
   3, score 6
   4, score 12
2. Add scores in each column to get column total.
3. Divide each column total by 6 to get column average.
4. Plot average scores for each intelligence on next page to make a bar graph.

L	M	L/M	S	B/K	IRP	IAP
		1 ___		2 ___		
			3 ___			4 ___
				5 ___		
		6 ___				
7 ___						8 ___
				9 ___		
			10 ___			
11 ___					12 ___	
			13 ___			
	14 ___		15 ___			
16 ___		17 ___				18 ___
					19 ___	
	20 ___	21 ___				
		22 ___				
	23 ___		24 ___	25 ___		
26 ___				27 ___	28 ___	29 ___
					30 ___	
31 ___						32 ___
	33 ___					
	34 ___				35 ___	
				36 ___		37 ___
					38 ___	
		39 ___				
	40 ___					
41 ___			42 ___			
TOTAL	TOTAL	TOTAL	TOTAL	TOTAL	TOTAL	TOTAL
___	___	___	___	___	___	___
AVERAGE	AVERAGE	AVERAGE	AVERAGE	AVERAGE	AVERAGE	AVERAGE
___	___	___	___	___	___	___

TABLE 4.5
(continued)

Multiple Intelligences Profile Indicator

Directions:
Graph the average score for each domain of intelligence. Darken between the
lines to create a bar graph. The longest bars indicate areas of primary strength of
operation. The medium-length bars indicate areas of supporting strength.

```
LINGUISTIC    ──────────────────────────────────────────────
              |   |   |   |   |   |   |   |   |   |    |    |
              0   1   2   3   4   5   6   7   8   9   10   11   12

MUSICAL       ──────────────────────────────────────────────
              |   |   |   |   |   |   |   |   |   |    |    |
              0   1   2   3   4   5   6   7   8   9   10   11   12

LOGICAL/
MATHEMA-      ──────────────────────────────────────────────
TICAL         |   |   |   |   |   |   |   |   |   |    |    |
              0   1   2   3   4   5   6   7   8   9   10   11   12

SPATIAL       ──────────────────────────────────────────────
              |   |   |   |   |   |   |   |   |   |    |    |
              0   1   2   3   4   5   6   7   8   9   10   11   12

BODILY/
KINESTHE-     ──────────────────────────────────────────────
TIC           |   |   |   |   |   |   |   |   |   |    |    |
              0   1   2   3   4   5   6   7   8   9   10   11   12

INTER-
PERSONAL      ──────────────────────────────────────────────
              |   |   |   |   |   |   |   |   |   |    |    |
              0   1   2   3   4   5   6   7   8   9   10   11   12

INTRA-
PERSONAL      ──────────────────────────────────────────────
              |   |   |   |   |   |   |   |   |   |    |    |
              0   1   2   3   4   5   6   7   8   9   10   11   12

              LOW....................................................HIGH
                        STRENGTH OF OPERATION
```

Source: Multiple Intelligence Profile Indicator based on the theory of Multiple
Intelligences by Howard Gardner, included with permission by author Frank Rainey,
consultant Colorado Dept. of Education, 1992.

verse and solving problems therein. One advantage to this element of self-discovery is that we can orchestrate projects and learning situations that minimize frustration, thereby enhancing personal pleasure and the probability of successful outcomes.

Creating business, educational, or recreational situations that are compatible with your intellectual domains will significantly reduce stress in your life.

5

Finding the Balance

There has been some concern about the great thinker, Democritus, the first person to conceive of the atomic structure of the universe. He had been observed sitting in the Public Square for days on end, apparently lost in thought. Concerned citizens called in Hippocrates, the town doctor. Well, the report is that he had examined Democritus and the worry is over. It turns out Democritus is actually stimulating his creativity by living inside his mind. Just a little meditation. Apparently when you are lost in thought some of your best ideas can be found.

—Daniel Goleman, Paul Kaufman, Michael Ray

The Creative Spirit

Understanding some basic psychological truths about ourselves is every bit as important as dealing with physiological factors like stress. In fact, as we'll see, it's often when our conscious version of ourselves is at odds with our not-so-freely-acknowledged wishes and desires that stress can set in. Moreover, many self-soothing techniques simply will not work unless we take an honest inventory of our values, behaviors, and attitudes. When there is harmony between our inner and outer worlds, then creativity—the deep-seated source of enduring pleasure and fulfillment—becomes manifest.

One of the greatest sources of inner turmoil is being out of sync with the guiding principles of one's life—when there is discord between an individual's conception of the desirable ends and means of action and her or his own patterns of behavior. If, for example, a person has high regard for a sense of accomplishment and finds that he or she has little to claim in the area of personal achievement, that person might well experience a chronic sense of dissatisfaction and discomfort, that is, stress.

Values: The Principles That Guide Your Life

Milton Rokeach and Sandra J. Ball-Rokeach of the University of Southern California have rigorously studied the role of values in people's lives. The Rokeach Value Survey, first published in 1967, was designed with the anticipation that it would provide information about individual and societal values. During the past twenty-five years, the survey has been widely used to assess how guiding principles are related to patterns of behavior.

> Two sets of 18 conceptions of the desirable are presented in alphabetical order. The first set represents terminal values, or the ultimate end goals of existence, such as wisdom, equality, peace or family security. The second set represents instrumental values, or the behavioral means for achieving such end goals, for instance the importance of being honest, ambitious, forgiving, or logical. The total number of such instrumental and terminal values is assumed to be relatively small; there are just so many end goals and just so many ideal modes of behavior for achieving them.

The items are presented alphabetically, with the instruction to arrange them in order of perceived importance, by assigning a rank of 1 to 18 for each of the two sets of values (i.e., eighteen instrumental values and eighteen terminal values). This process takes about fifteen to twenty minutes for adults and has been successfully accomplished by people ranging in age from eleven to ninety. Readers are now invited to rank, and therefore prioritize, the guiding principles of their lives (terminal values) and the relative importance of personal qualities and standards of conduct (instrumental values). The Rokeach terminal and instrumental values are shown in Table 5.1.

A national sample of American adults was asked to rank the values as shown in Table 5.1. Over a sixteen-year study period, from 1968 to 1984, American terminal values were shown to have remained remarkably stable; that is, the top and bottom six values remained almost entirely unchanged, and not one of the six top and bottom items varied by more than one rank in any of the four national surveys taken during the study period.

As of 1984, Americans prioritized their top six terminal values as (1) Family Security, (2) A World of Peace, (3) Freedom, (4) Self-Respect, (5) Happiness, and (6) Wisdom. The six values that were

TABLE 5.1

Rokeach Value Inventory

(A) Terminal Values	Rank Order
A comfortable life (a prosperous life)	————
Equality (brotherhood, equal opportunity for all)	————
An exciting life (a stimulating, active life)	————
Family security (taking care of loved ones)	————
Freedom (independence, free choice)	————
Happiness (contentedness)	————
Inner Harmony (freedom from inner conflict)	————
Mature love (sexual and spiritual intimacy)	————
National security (protection from attack)	————
Pleasure (an enjoyable, leisurely life)	————
Salvation (saved, eternal life)	————
Self-respect (self-esteem)	————
Sense of accomplishment (lasting contribution)	————
Social recognition (respect, admiration)	————
True friendship (close companionship)	————
Wisdom (a mature understanding of life)	————
A world of beauty (beauty of nature and the arts)	————
A world at peace (free of war and conflict)	————

(B) Instrumental Values	
Ambitious (hard-working, aspiring)	————
Broadminded (open-minded)	————
Capable (competent, effective)	————
Cheerful (lighthearted, joyful)	————
Clean (neat, tidy)	————
Courageous (standing up for your beliefs)	————
Forgiving (willing to pardon others)	————
Helpful (working for the welfare of others)	————
Honest (sincere, truthful)	————
Imaginative (daring, creative)	————
Independent (self-reliant, self-sufficient)	————
Intellectual (intelligent, reflective)	————
Logical (consistent, rational)	————
Loving (affectionate, tender)	————
Obedient (dutiful, respectful)	————
Polite (courteous, well-mannered)	————
Responsible (dependable, reliable)	————
Self-controlled (restrained, self-disciplined)	————

ranked as least important were (12) Equality, (13) National Security, (14) Mature Love, (15) A World of Beauty, (16) Pleasure, (17) An Exciting Life, and (18) Social Recognition.

Available data on the ranking of instrumental values show a similar pattern of stability. The top-ranking instrumental values were (1) Honest, (2) Ambitious, (3) Responsible, (4) Forgiving, (5) Broad-Minded, and (6) Courageous. The instrumental values that received the lowest priorities were (12) Independent, (13) Cheerful, (14) Polite, (15) Intelligent, (16) Obedient, (17) Logical, (18) Imaginative.

Although the Rokeaches were impressed by the apparent stability of American values, they regard change in prioritization of Equality (brotherhood and equal opportunity for all) as particularly significant. In 1971, Americans ranked Equality as fourth, while in 1981, Equality slipped in priority to twelfth. There were also noticeable increases in personal values, showing greater emphasis on A Comfortable Life and A Sense of Accomplishment and Excitement. At the same time, there was a decline in the ranking of National Security. Another interesting finding concerns the value of A World of Beauty:

> Young people start out with a natural appreciation of beauty. But in the process of growing up we somehow knock this sense of appreciation out of them. Eleven year-olds rank A World of Beauty seventh in importance . . . and by the time they reach adulthood A World of Beauty has plummeted . . . down the list to 17th in importance.

The societal values of the 1990s are yet to be described. Most likely, they will not vary radically from those reported during the past two decades.

At this point, the reader is asked to consider his or her personal values. Can you attribute personal stress to a discrepancy between your own values and your actual behavior? What tension may be produced by the relative importance you place on particular ends and means versus the values of those around you? The implications are clear: if dissatisfaction exists, a person may contemplate changing his or her values, behavior, or even society at large. Confronting these discrepancies is consistent with the tradition set forth by John Dewey, who said, "Thinking begins with a felt difficulty," and also with the wisdom of Benjamin Franklin: "The things which hurt instruct."

Identifying Your Pleasure Orientations

A secret of attaining prolonged pleasure is to integrate an array of enjoyable activities with the values that guide our existence. All too often, however, we remain largely unaware of not only our value priorities, but even the very activities we find enjoyable. By bringing our pleasure orientations to the forefront of awareness, we increase the likelihood of achieving a balance between what we deem important and the things we actually do.

Kenneth Wanberg and one of the authors of this book (Milkman) have classified the kinds of activities from which human beings derive pleasure. After having administered the Personal Pleasure Inventory (PPI) to a diverse population of several hundred adults, Wanberg and Milkman have identified four broad pleasure dimensions:

1. Physical Expression
2. Self-Focus
3. Aesthetic Discovery
4. Collective Harmony

Each dimension is defined by a specific group of related activities. The dimension of *Physical Expression* includes Athletic Prowess and Challenging Nature. Within the broad dimension of *Self-Focus* are the factors of Physical Fitness, Sensuality, Soothing Sensations, and Material Comforts. The dimension of *Aesthetic Discovery* includes Artistic Seeking Adventure, Experiencing Nature, Domestic Involvement, Reflective Relaxation, and Stimulation. *Collective Harmony* combines the factors of Mental Exercise, People Closeness, Religious Involvement, and Altruistic Interests. Pleasure orientations are not mutually exclusive; that is, aesthetic appreciation of music and art may coincide with pleasurable stimulation derived from learning to play a musical instrument, combined with joy from playing with others.

Readers are invited to complete an abbreviated version of the PPI, as shown in Table 5.2. The scoring system allows respondents to measure themselves on the fifteen aforementioned pleasure orientations. By focusing on the activities from which you and your associates derive pleasure, you can not only communicate more openly about your needs and desires, but also pursue a more goal-directed

TABLE 5.2

Personal Pleasure Inventory (PPI), Abbreviated Form

Instructions

0 = Never engaged in activity or no pleasure derived from activity
1 = Low degree of pleasure derived
2 = Moderate degree of pleasure derived
3 = High degree of pleasure derived
4 = Very high degree of pleasure derived

Using the above key, please rate the following items as to degree of pleasure that you derived from each activity. Place the appropriate number corresponding to your choice in the blank line opposite the item. Then put the total score for each group of items on the line marked Total for Scale.

1. Athletic Prowess
   _____ Playing basketball.
   _____ Playing tennis.
   _____ Watching sports.
   _____ Playing softball.
   _____ Going to football games.
   _____ Playing golf.
   _____ Playing football and soccer.
   _____ Playing volleyball.
   _____ TOTAL FOR SCALE 1

2. Challenging Nature
   _____ Floating on a raft.
   _____ Canoeing.
   _____ White-water rafting.
   _____ Camping out.
   _____ Hiking.
   _____ Skiing.
   _____ TOTAL FOR SCALE 2

3. Physical Fitness
   _____ Eating healthy foods.
   _____ Exercising.
   _____ Biking.
   _____ Stretching.
   _____ Walking.
   _____ TOTAL FOR SCALE 3

4. Sensuality
   _____ Making love.
   _____ Kissing and cuddling.
   _____ Giving flowers to your lover.

TABLE 5.2
(continued)

_____ Erotic sex.
_____ Going to the beach.
_____ TOTAL FOR SCALE 4

5. Soothing Sensations
   _____ Listening to soft music.
   _____ Warming self by fire.
   _____ Soaking in hot tub.
   _____ Having back rubbed.
   _____ Massage.
   _____ Eating in nice restaurant.
   _____ TOTAL FOR SCALE 5

6. Material Comforts
   _____ Making money.
   _____ Shopping.
   _____ Spending money.
   _____ Going out for an evening.
   _____ Improving outward appearance.
   _____ TOTAL FOR SCALE 6

7. Seeking Adventure
   _____ Driving to new places.
   _____ Visiting different cities.
   _____ Experiencing new places.
   _____ Experiencing new things.
   _____ Traveling to foreign cities.
   _____ Visiting different cultures.
   _____ TOTAL FOR SCALE 7

8. Experiencing Nature
   _____ Being in nature.
   _____ Being in the woods.
   _____ Watching wildlife.
   _____ Watching the stars.
   _____ Watching the sun rise.
   _____ TOTAL FOR SCALE 8

9. Domestic Involvement
   _____ Redecorating home.
   _____ Remodeling home.
   _____ Working on home projects.
   _____ Painting house.
   _____ Gardening.
   _____ TOTAL FOR SCALE 9

TABLE 5.2

(continued)

10. Reflective Relaxation
    _____ Meditation.
    _____ Relaxation exercises.
    _____ Daily meditations.
    _____ Self-reflection.
    _____ Journal writing.
    _____ TOTAL FOR SCALE 10

11. Artistic Stimulation
    _____ Going to the theater.
    _____ Attending symphony.
    _____ Creating artwork.
    _____ Reading books.
    _____ Writing poetry/fiction.
    _____ Playing musical instrument.
    _____ TOTAL FOR SCALE 11

12. Mental Exercise
    _____ Word games.
    _____ Playing cards.
    _____ Crossword puzzles.
    _____ Solving mystery games.
    _____ Sewing.
    _____ TOTAL FOR SCALE 12

13. People Closeness
    _____ Helping family members.
    _____ Playing with children.
    _____ Being with family.
    _____ Being with friends.
    _____ Hugging.
    _____ Being with a partner.
    _____ TOTAL FOR SCALE 13

14. Religious Involvement
    _____ Spiritual thinking.
    _____ Worship.
    _____ Bible study.
    _____ Church work.
    _____ Going to church.
    _____ Praying.
    _____ TOTAL FOR SCALE 14

TABLE 5.2
(continued)

---

15. Altruistic Efforts
    _____ Counseling others.
    _____ Helping others.
    _____ Teaching others.
    _____ Volunteering services.
    _____ Writing letters to friends or family.
    _____ TOTAL FOR SCALE 15

When you have finished scoring all of your responses, place the Total Score for each scale on the profile in the appropriate box (opposite page) under the Raw Score column. Then find the corresponding raw score on the row for that particular scale to determine your percentile rank for that scale. The percentile rank indicates the degree of pleasure that you derive from each orientation compared with that derived by others. For example, if your raw score for Material Comforts is 17, then you enjoy this pleasure orientation more than 80% of the sample population do, which is roughly typical of a mixed group of college-educated adults.

---

pathway to pleasure. Are your values and daily activities consistent with the pleasure centers you have identified? Can you strengthen or improve intimacy by sharing activities that are mutually enjoyable?

Adjusting Your Attitude

"Hey, man, you got an attitude problem or what!"—this confrontational street vernacular may be the prelude to an argument, a fistfight, or even worse. On a less sensational level, your state of mind relative to people, objects, and events can have positive or negative effects on work, love, and play. There is mounting evidence that *optimism* is a powerful antidote to the harmful effects of stress.

Now that you have a better grasp of some of the values and attitudes that determine how you deal with everyday situations, it may be simpler for you to take the optimism option.

David Sobel, coauthor of *The Healing Brain and Healthy Pleasures,* discusses how attitudes and beliefs are typically viewed as precursors of whether or not people will engage in positive health practices. More important, however, is the finding that beliefs and

Personal Pleasure Inventory Primary Scales

NAME_____ DATE_____ AGENCY_____

GENDER [ ] MALE [ ] FEMALE   AGE_____   I.D. NO._____

	SCALE NAME	RAW SCORE	_{1\} 1	2	3	4	5	6	7	8	9	10
PHY / EXP	1. ATHLETIC PROWESS		0 2 3 4	5 6 7	8 9 10	11 12	13	14 15	16 17	18 19 20	21 22 23	24 26 32
	2. CHALLENGING NATURE		0 2 3 5	6 7	8	9 10	11 12	13	14 15	16 17	18 19	20 21 24
SELF FOCUS	3. PHYSICAL FITNESS		2 5 6 7	8	10	11		12	13	14	15	16 18 20
	4. SENSUALITY		1 6 8 9	10 11 12	13	14	15	16	17	18		19 20
	5. SOOTHING SENSATIONS		4 10 11	12 13 14	15	16	17	18	19	20	21 22	23 24
	6. MATERIAL COMFORTS		4 7 8 9	10 11	12	13	14	15	16	17	18	19 20
AESTHETIC DISCOVERY	7. SEEKING ADVENTURE		4 7 8 9	10 11 12	13	14 15	16	17 18	19	20 21	22	23 24
	8. EXPERIENCING NATURE		1 6 7 8	9 10	11	12	13	14	15	16 17	18	19 20
	9. DOMESTIC INVOLVEMENT		0 1 2	3	4	5 6	7	8	9	10	11 12 13	14 15 19
	10. REFLECTIVE RELAXATION		0 1 2	3	4	5	6	7	8	9 10	11 12	13 15 20
	11. ARTISTIC STIMULATION		0 2 3	4 5 6	7	8	9	10 11	12	13 14	15 16 17	18 20 24
COLLECTIVE HARMONY	12. MENTAL EXERCISE		0 1 2	3 4	5	6	7		8	9	10 11	12 14 20
	13. PEOPLE CLOSENESS		4 11 12	13 14	15 16	17	18	19	20	21	22	23 24
	14. RELIGIOUS INVOLVEMENT		0	1	2	3	4 5	6	7 8	9 10	11 12	13 14 15 16 19 24
	15. ALTRUISTIC EFFORTS		1 6 7	8	9	10	11	12	13	14	15	16 17 20

DECILE RANK (columns 1–10)

PERCENTILE: 1 · 10 · 20 · 30 · 40 · 50 · 60 · 70 · 80 · 90 · 99

attitudes have their own specific effects. There are direct pathways between optimism or pessimism and health outcomes, including the extent of your physical, emotional, intellectual, and spiritual well-being.

In a talk entitled "The Optimism Antidote: When Belief Becomes Biology," Sobel describes how a positive outlook allowed him to gain control over a childhood illness that he found to be chronically embarrassing and stressful. David Sobel suffered from warts from ages eight to eleven. He describes late childhood as a period during which he was "cut up, frozen, injected with toxic agents, and painted with lethal chemicals." Nothing worked. At one point during his desperate struggle, he came across an article entitled "Warts Cured by Suggestion," so he thought, "Tell the warts to go away!" He repeated the phrase "Warts, go away" ten times each day, and after two weeks, lo and behold, they were gone.

Paralleling Sobel's amazing childhood discovery, medical science has produced substantial evidence that the mind can, in fact, exert powerful influence over the body. It can regulate the flow of blood; the course of viruses, such as those that cause warts; and the immune system in general. In a British study first published by Sinclair-Gieber et al. in *Lancet* (1959), nine of fourteen patients with warts responded positively to the suggestion that warts on one side of their body would regress. After reviewing fifteen studies with a total of 1,000 patients, Sobel found that one-third of the patients who are given a positive suggestion will experience relief in such diverse health matters as seasickness, postoperative wound pain, hypertension, angina, asthma, hay fever, and acne. In short, no body system is immune to the effect of an optimistic attitude.

In a classic study of a woman with intractable nausea and vomiting, Stuart Wolfe preceded administering medicine with the suggestion, "We have this powerful medicine that can cure you." He then gathered objective data on the extent of her peristaltic contractions, showing that her condition had markedly improved. In fact, Wolfe and his colleagues had administered syrup of ipecac—a powerful emetic used to induce vomiting!

In another dramatic demonstration of the power of belief over biology, Hank Bennett, a psychologist at the University of California at Davis, recognized how little time doctors afforded their patients while preparing them for surgery. He observed that the doctors seemed to spend more time washing their hands than advising people how to manage the strain of going under the knife. Bennett decided to test his idea that mental preparation—specifically, the suggestion that patients could control their postoperative blood loss—might have beneficial effects. Bennett varied the preoperative instructions to three groups of surgery patients: group 1 had standard medical preparation; group 2 was given basic relaxation training; and group 3 was given the instruction "When someone says something embarrassing, you blush. [Obviously, the mind has control over the automatic responses of the body.] During surgery I want you to close down the arteries around your spine and after I want you to return blood for healing." The researchers found an average blood loss during surgery of 900 cubic centimeters in the first two groups. Experimental patients in group 3, however, showed an average blood loss of only 500 cubic centimeters. These findings are significant because, whereas the first two groups did require the unwelcome procedure of blood transfusion, the experimental group did not.

In addition to positive suggestion, Sobel found that by helping people to develop optimism—a belief that things might very well go their way—they were more likely to succeed across all categories of human endeavor. In nearly every case, positive expectations about the outcome of a major life event could be fostered by professionals becoming sensitized to the nuances in how they communicated with a person under their care. In terminal illness, for example, consider the effect of the following prognostic reports: (1) 80 percent of patients with this type of cancer die, while (2) 20 percent of these patients are survivors—you can be one of the latter.

Other crucial stimuli for anticipating the unknown with positivity are *enthusiasm* and *feedback*. In a study of dental patients, one group was told, "Here is a medication that can relieve pain and anxiety. I feel very positive about this treatment." Another group was told, "Here is a pill that has worked for some patients, but I have seen little success in my practice"—and rated their pain and anxiety much higher than the first group did. People also benefit from being told how they are doing—from being given feedback—along the way of a difficult undertaking, task, or journey. Soldiers, for examples, who participated in a long march did their best when they were given constant reports about their progress during each phase of their assignment.

Optimism is also predicated on self-efficacy, the belief in one's ability to have a positive impact on a situation or event. Albert Bandura has shown that people who are confident about their ability to succeed are in fact more likely to do so. Few Olympic gold medalists believe they qualify "only" for a silver or bronze. A major factor in self-confidence is the degree to which people perceive they have control over their own fate. Arthritis patients who received information from lay leaders about the impact of nutrition and other health practices experienced a 20 percent decrease in their symptoms, about as good as with anti-inflammatory medication. When Kate Lorig of Stanford University interviewed arthritis patients who did not get better, she identified a shared belief that there was nothing they could do to control their illness. With significant success, Lorig and her colleagues then changed the program to enhance patients' sense of control, confidence, and efficacy.

The findings are unequivocal: optimism is a significant ally as we strive for optimal health and well-being throughout the lifespan. Sobel found that self-reported health is a better predictor of future mortality than doctors' predictions, often based on high-tech data analysis. Health optimists live longer than health pessimists. When other risk/resiliency factors are held constant (i.e., when people are matched for exercise, nutrition, drug use, etc.), aside from age, health optimism is the greatest predictor of longevity. It follows that there are few questions of greater relevance than how we can promote optimism in ourselves and the people around us whom we care for and love.

Martin Seligman and Chris Peterson of the University of Pennsylvania developed a model of optimism based on how we interpret life events. Optimists explain things differently. Consider, for example, the scenario when you come home, dog-tired after a hard day at work, only to find that your spouse has walked out on you. Was it something *you* did, or something *your partner* did? Is it likely to *continue,* or will it *get better*? Does it affect only the relationship with your *spouse,* or everything *else* you do? Seligman has shown that pessimists have internal, stable, and global explanatory styles (e.g., "It's my fault"; "It won't improve"; and "It will screw up my entire life").

When Seligman investigated the attributions (explanatory styles) of Hall of Fame baseball players by reviewing their published explanations and predictions regarding world events, he found that pessimists have shorter lives. Harvard graduates from nineteen to thirty-nine who revealed themselves to be pessimists in interviews during the time of their graduation showed higher mortality and disease rates years later. All of this suggests that the stories we use to explain the world around us may determine how long we live and how much fun we have while we're here.

The first step of self-improvement in this area is to track your thoughts when you notice a negative emotional state. Consider accidentally meeting an old flame, then feeling downhearted and tense. It may turn out that the story you are telling yourself runs something like this: "I'm getting old; I'll never have any more romance; I'm no longer attractive to the opposite sex." Obviously, the story you are telling yourself is intimately related to the depression you now feel. The skill is to examine the tales that surround your negative feelings, and begin to refute them. Sobel suggests the following inventory for discovering whether *style of thinking* is at the root of your unhappiness. Are you

- thinking in all-or-none terms?
- generalizing from one situation to another?
- assigning too much probability to rare events?
- overlooking your strengths?
- blaming yourself for not being in control of something that you could not possibly control?
- getting caught up in shortsighted dramas, rather than considering what difference this will make in days, weeks or years?

Cognitive psychologists have shown that by giving serious consideration to these questions, we can shift our style of thinking from negative to positive. And what is there to lose? Even if optimists don't really live longer, have fewer colds, cure herpes, or boost their immune system, they still reap a windfall of benefits by improving their quality of life—and that's nothing to sneeze at. All of this, of course, is not to diminish the wisdom of heeding sound medical advice. When the Dalai Lama was asked what he thought about the popular concept of New Age guilt (i.e., "What bad thoughts or previous misdeeds are the cause of your illness?", he responded, "Don't these people know about bacteria, viruses, and biochemical disturbances?"

Imagination: Blessing or Curse

Jerome Singer of Yale University is renowned for his research and theorizing on the adaptive role of imagination. He proposes that fantasy can be described as "the ability to reproduce faces of persons, snatches of dialogue or objects no longer immediately available to the primary senses and then to reshape further the memories of these experiences into new and complex forms."

The basic function of imagery is to explore our relationship to the world. We develop specific mental pictures of who we are, which become a kind of personal identity uniting our past experiences to our intended actions. By imagining, we can work through painful memories and sufferings or formulate models of enchantment through which we will soar to blissful heights with our lovers, family, or friends.

The emergence of new ideas from the reshaping of a multiplicity of past events becomes, in a sense, a vast additional source of knowledge. Fantasy, the wellspring of creativity, may be thought of as a piece of God. In this regard, Albert Einstein remarked, "When I examine myself and my methods of thought, I come to the conclusion the gift of fantasy has meant more to me than my talent for absorbing positive knowledge."

Whereas fairy tales provide fantasy guideposts for children to master the tasks of growing up, religion and myths provide ethical prescriptions for conduct in the adult world. The adaptive function of imagination, however, far exceeds that of helping to establish meaning, purpose, and patterns of conduct in an often confusing existence. Fantasy affords us an internal system for reducing stress. We can diminish tension through the imagined gratification of physical or psychological impulses. By creating alternative mental environments, we are temporarily released from internal conflict or from tension in the outside world. By virtue of these intense reward capabilities, we regularly rely on fantasy solutions to everyday problems in living.

In fact, moderate use of imagination is necessary for adaptive living. Personality research with overeaters and drug abusers, for example, reveals their impoverished fantasy lives. These people often react as if they respond only to external stimulation. The outside world seems to cry out, "Take me! Swallow me! Feed me! Hug me!" Similarly, children who do not partake of imagination play tend more toward fighting, delinquency, and antisocial acts.

There is ample evidence that the imagery system is tied not only to more or less adaptive patterns of behavior, but to physical health as well. Obviously, as shown in Chapter 3, if you are in a real danger or stress situation, your body reacts chemically at the level of the autonomic and central nervous system. Singer finds that frightening or hostile fantasies have similar effects:

Suppose you are not in the actual situation, but you are a guilty daydream type and you imagine yourself having betrayed your friend and having to be on trial . . . or standing at the gates of heaven before St. Peter and having to explain to him how you betrayed him or were cruel to him and so on. Suddenly you *are* in that situation. Or if you have frightening fantasies as some people have, of the atom bomb landing on your town, and this comes back for you, again and again. You are temporarily in that situation and you are providing the same type of physical response.

Research shows that dire consequences may be associated with excessive fantasies that involve either fear or anger. In a study conducted at Yale University, Singer found that people who showed an excess of "conscious, angry, hostile fantasies" were more likely to have hypertensive responses and aroused blood pressure as a natural reaction not just when they were having a fantasy, but as a consistent physiological pattern. While some theorize that it's good for people to fantasize in order to release their aggression, Singer concludes that generally it's *not* good to be angry. In fact, we should strive to find situations that avoid anger.

> There are times where [controlled expression of] anger is essential to communicate effectively with other people, but if you can work out your life in such a way that you don't have to be angry much of the time, it would be much better for you . . . [H]ostile and aggressive thoughts and fantasies create a negative kind of body feedback which can have damaging consequences.

The message is clear: keep an eye on your anger because it can make you sick. Repressing hostility is not good, either. Research shows that those who are unaware of their deep-seated angry feelings are prone to certain forms of cancer. Singer finds that "the angry fantasies of the cardiovascular people are creating one problem; the happy fantasies—or denial—of the repressors are creating another problem." The direction for health and well-being is to steer clear of anger-eliciting circumstances and, when this is impossible, to responsibly express and acknowledge how you feel.

Redford Williams, author of *The Trusting Heart* and professor of psychiatry at Duke University, suggests twelve steps for reducing hostility and associated heart disease. As shown in Table 5.3, the first step is to monitor your cynical thoughts with a "Hostility Log." The remaining steps follow in logical sequence.

TABLE 5.3
Reducing Hostility

When you wish to reduce hostility, the most important first step to achieve this goal is to begin to measure your hostile behaviors. All that is required is a small, pocket-sized notebook that can be carried in a shirt pocket at all times. Whenever you become aware of cynical thoughts, angry feelings, or aggressive behaviors that you are experiencing or emitting, note them down according to the following format:

When:

Where:

Who: [Here note the identity of the person who stimulated the thoughts, feelings, and/or behaviors.]

What: [Here note what the other person did.]

Thoughts: [Here note the content of your thoughts.]

Feelings: [Here describe the feelings you experienced, whether emotion (e.g., anger, annoyance) or physical (e.g., heart pounding, breath short).]

Actions: [Here describe what you actually did.]

After two weeks of keeping your Hostility Log, you will begin to recognize your hostility at increasingly early points in the "hostility cascade" from cynical thoughts to angry feelings to aggressive acts. This will enable you to apply the other steps that I suggest to short-circuit your hostility before it can gather momentum and begin to do you emotional and physical harm.

- Confess your hostility to yourself and a confidant and seek help to change
- Stop cynical thoughts
- Reason with yourself
- Put yourself in the other person's shoes
- Laugh at yourself
- Learn to relax
- Force yourself to trust others
- Force yourself to listen more
- Substitute assertiveness for aggression
- Pretend today is your last
- Practice forgiveness

Dream Work

If one advances in the direction of his dreams, one will meet with success unexpected in common hours.

—Henry David Thoreau

To be sure, when our thoughts focus on anger, hostility, or pain, imagination is a kind of curse, intensifying the suffering that already exists. On counterpoint, however, fantasy can serve as a lifeline to optimal living. In the classic book *Man and His Symbols,* Carl Jung discusses how dream images are psychic gifts that may be used as invaluable resources for solving major life problems. According to Jung's theory, nearly all dreams are compensatory—they point toward what is missing in the dreamer's attitude or lifestyle, elements that, when properly attended to, will result in improved health and well-being. Often the dream represents a view that is opposite to the actual life situation of the dreamer. The purpose of this contradiction is to alert the dreamer to deficits or gaps in conscious experience. If the dreamer's self-image is low, the dream may try to lift it up. On the other hand, if one's self-evaluation is too high, the dream may serve as a reminder that certain attitudes or behaviors need improvement.

Ira Progoff, who studied directly with Jung in Zurich, has developed techniques for making constructive use of dreams and other elements of imagination. He recommends utilization of the "dream log," wherein dreams are recorded as accurately as possible, with no amplification whatsoever. Later, you can extend the dream process by reentering the dream, through a technique Progoff refers to as "twilight imagery." You put yourself back into the dream and "feel" the process, avoiding becoming lost in trying to find the dream's secret meaning and instead becoming open to the quality and tone of the dream and allowing its message to come through. You can write in the "dream enlargement" section of your journal whatever comes to you.

The entire dream process can be compared to a train journey, except that we do not know the destination in advance. The ride may be frightening as we glimpse unpleasant places, but these are only tunnels en route to self-discovery. According to Progoff, "We can discover the destination of our dreams and can recognize that the destination often contains the goal and meaning of our life unfoldment as a whole."

Dreaming always contains the seed of the process of self-discovery, and the process can be derailed by overanalysis. Progoff suggests working, if possible, with a series of dreams, focusing on the ones that tend to draw you in the most. If you feel that a dream has a message to give you, write it down. By getting down to the twilight level to extend the process of dreaming, "we find that many inner awarenessess about our life, our past and the possibilities about our futures are actively stimulated." After you have recorded these awarenesses in the dream journal, you can think about them with clarity.

> Many new thoughts, insights, intuitions and recognitions of all kinds related to our life in general and to specific projects now come to our mind. Sometimes they come to consciousness in great volume, flooding us with ideas and awarenesses. At such times we have to learn to regulate their flow so that we can retain and record them.

Progoff has developed the method of "Intensive Journal Writing" for becoming actively involved in discovering the movement and meaning of your life. Distinctly different from a diary, Progoff's method provides a multilevel feedback system that integrates conscious and unconscious fantasies, gently unfolding the meaning and purpose of one's life. "The goal of journal writing is neither literary creation nor religious soul-searching, but an active self-transforming involvement."

Readers are invited to adopt the guidelines, as shown in Table 5.4, for utilizing the amazing gift of fantasy to improve self-understanding and personal intimacy—in Progoff's words, "to make the world a gentler place and to become aware of those subtle intonations of truth that give direction to our lives." According to Anaïs Nin, a diarist who logged more than 150,000 pages, "The lack of intimacy with one's self and consequently with others is what created the loneliest and most alienated people in the world."

Progoff's techniques represent a synthesis of Jungian psychology and shamanic methods of dream interpretation that have been practiced for centuries across time, place, and culture. Shamanic Journeying, an ancient technique utilized by the healers of many Native

TABLE 5.4
The Way of the Journal

- Where are you now in your life? Form an image.
- Recapitulations and Rememberings—quick, significant scenes in our lives.
- Stepping Stones—important events or people captured in a word or two or an image.
- Intersections—Roads Taken and Not Taken.
- Twilight Imagery—Turn your attention inward and wait in stillness and let yourself observe the various forms of imagery that present themselves.
- Dialogue Dimension—Engage in imaginary conversations with some of the significant people already listed in the Stepping Stone section. Go through a short Stepping Stone exercise for the "other." After the exercise, reread what you have written and write down how you feel.

American tribes, incorporates the use of deep-breathing and relaxation techniques, drumming, and waking dreaming. These waking dreams are out-of-body journeys that occur when the journeyer is totally aware of his or her body in the physical world and is also aware of being inside the dream. The journeyer begins in a darkened, quiet room by lying down in a comfortable position and covering him- or herself with a warm blanket. As with transcendental meditation, the body's metabolism is slowed and body temperature is slightly lowered. The shaman smudges the area and the journeyer with sage to purify the space. The journeyer then begins deep breathing and focusing on relaxing specific areas of the body until all tension is released.

The shaman begins drumming (or playing an audiotape of drumming), utilizing a steady, repetitious rhythm. The journeyer enters what Michael Harner, author of *The Way of the Shaman,* calls the Shamanic State of Consciousness (SSC).

> The SSC involves not only a "trance" or a transcendent state of awareness, but also a learned awareness of shamanic methods and assumptions while in such an altered state. . . . the SSC is the cognitive condition in which one perceives the "nonordinary reality" of Carlos Castaneda, and the "extraordinary manifestations of reality" of Robert Lowie.

The journeyer begins by envisioning a natural opening in the earth—a hot spring, puddle, lake, ocean, cave, and so on. The journeyer "enters" the opening and "travels" down a tunnel to the Lowerworld—the world existing below our everyday reality, in essence, the subconscious. While in the Lowerworld, the journeyer has as a purpose the resolving of ordinary conflicts, through interaction with the entities encountered there—animals, humans, and "spirits."

Michelle Redifer, a thirty-four-year-old incest survivor, had been studying Native American spirituality for a few years before she began retrieving the memories of her abuse by her long-deceased father. She found that entering into a dialogue with her dream entities provided her with the necessary outlet for her rage and empowered her with the emotional tools that initiated the healing process.

> I needed more help than therapy alone could provide—something that combined my strong Native spiritual beliefs with traditional psychology. A close friend knew of my work with a Lakota medicine man and suggested I study Journeying with her friend Tony Arguello, an apprenticing shaman for twelve years and traditional mental health professional. Tony had experienced great success with his incest clients through the use of Shamanic Journeying and soul retrieval.
>
> My family was extremely dysfunctional; I've been able to trace incest and other forms of abuse through six generations. Therefore, I didn't feel safe enough to turn to my family for support in the initial stages of my healing. I had unethical or apathetic encounters with three mental health professionals and distrusted the traditional psychological approach. For me, Journeying combined the best elements of traditional and spiritual therapy.
>
> By becoming "empowered" by my animal and spirit allies, I achieved a place of safety and comfort that enabled me to confront my father mentally. I could vent my extreme rage at him—sometimes verbally, sometimes physically—in a safe, controlled environment. I was also able to connect with and comfort myself at various ages, thus retrieving fragmented pieces of my soul or spirit. I envisioned holding myself at six, eleven, and sixteen years of age and offering my "child" comfort and protection.
>
> My Journeying encounters were so vivid that I found myself compelled to keep a journal of my experiences. Soon, my journal entries evolved into a metaphoric nonfiction story of my incest. I chose the natural conflict between sheep ranchers and coyotes to represent the incest perpetrators and victims. All of the animal characters I encoun-

tered in my Journeying have found their way into my book chronicling my healing—an assertive badger, a courageous bear, a nurturing turtle, a gentle deer, a transmuting snake, an edifying beaver, a guiding mountain lion, and a stealthy fox. After some time, I realized the animals represented my close friends and the lessons I had learned from them that facilitated my healing process and taught me how not to be a victim or abuser again—assertiveness, courage, gentleness, and leadership.

Actually, Progoff's concept of twilight imagery—putting oneself back into the dream, becoming open to its quality and tone, and allowing its message to come through—and the Shamanic Journey are quite similar. In both cases, healing takes place because the dreamer is allowed to explore the meaning of personal symbols, which carry vital directives and truths, through the safe reenactment and positive resolution of traumatic life events. Once the inner voyage is initiated, the dream becomes a self-directing healer. In this regard, Albert Schweitzer reportedly observed, "The witch doctor succeeds for the same reason all of the rest of us [doctors] succeed. Each patient carries his own doctor inside him. They come to us not knowing this truth. We are at our best when we give the doctor who resides within each patient a chance to go to work."

Increasing Personal Calm

Herbert Benson is chief of the Section on Behavioral Medicine at New England Deaconess Hospital and associate professor of medicine at Harvard Medical School. After completing medical training in cardiology, Benson became interested in how the mind affects the body, and particularly how high blood pressure might be influenced by emotional states. Benson was trying to gather scientific evidence for what had long been assumed in medical circles: that there is a positive correlation between stress and cardiovascular disease, and, further, that relaxation training could diminish the harmful effects of environmental threat. Colloquial expressions supporting his notion were commonplace: "Keep your cool—your blood pressure will go up"; "Don't get excited—you'll develop hypertension." In the late 1960s, Benson and his colleagues were able to show that certain environmental influences could, in fact, raise or lower blood pressure in a group of laboratory monkeys. Further, the monkeys could be trained to increase or decrease their blood pressure on cue.

One day in 1968, a group of young people came in to see Benson with a soft-spoken challenge:

Why are you fooling around with monkeys?
Why don't you study us?
We practice Transcendental Meditation.

Benson, reacting to his role as Harvard scientist, tried to dissuade the group. But they persisted. Finally, he decided that little would be lost by seeing whether or not there might be physiological changes attendant to the practice of transcendental meditation (TM). He and his colleagues brought healthy volunteers to the laboratory and had them sit for an entire hour, getting used to the instruments that would measure oxygen consumption—an index of the body's total metabolism—and carbon dioxide elimination—the amount of waste product that parallels oxygen usage. Measurements were taken in three twenty-minute intervals: (1) premeditation; (2) meditation—during which the subjects changed neither their posture nor their activity, only what they were thinking about; and (3) postmeditation—wherein subjects were instructed to go back to their regular mode of thinking.

Benson found a 16 to 17 percent decrease in oxygen consumption, with a parallel decrease in the amount of carbon dioxide elimination. This meant that by simply changing their thoughts, meditators could induce a significant change in their body's overall metabolism. The fact that the ratio of oxygen to carbon dioxide remained constant between the premeditation and meditation conditions showed that the meditators were neither breathing rapidly nor holding their breath to bring about the observed physiological changes. There was a true decrease in the overall amount of oxygen being used by the body. Correspondingly, during the meditation interval, there was a decrease of about two or three breaths per minute in rate of breathing (dropping from thirteen or fourteen breaths per minute to about eleven breaths). Subsequently, while studying advanced meditators in India, Benson and his colleagues were able to document respiratory rates as low as zero to one breath per minute for three to four minutes on end; the advanced meditators could so quiet their overall metabolism that they could, in effect, stop breathing. Further, there was no change in the arterial concentration of oxygen. The cells were getting enough oxygen; they were simply using less. There was also a precipitous fall in arterial blood lactate, high levels of which are associated with stress, anxiety, or disquietude, low levels with peace and tranquillity.

To his amazement, Benson documented some of the lowest levels of human metabolic activity ever recorded. At the time, there were only two physiological states known to cause these kind of changes: sleep and hibernation.

A hibernative animal shows a decrease in rectal temperature of two to three degrees, whereas a sleeping animal shows a change of only two-tenths to three-tenths of a degree. Incidentally, after sneaking into the den of some Alaskan grizzly bears and finding the animals sleeping while sitting up, two intrepid physiologists are said to have placed several quarts of maraschino cherries in front of one bear, which naturally, because of its love of sweet fruit, leaned forward. The investigators, taking advantage of the postural tilt, proceeded to make their measurements. The bear awoke, was understandably irate, and chased the investigators, who miraculously escaped unharmed, data in hand (so to speak). In fact, bears do not hibernate—they sleep.

Under much less hazardous conditions, Benson and his colleagues were able to show that meditation was not a hibernatory state. But the data could not be explained as a sleep state, either. The observed increase in alpha and theta wave frequencies were distinctly different from those which could be measured during ordinary sleep. Benson suspected that the changes brought about through TM were opposite to what had been described nearly three-quarters of a century earlier by Walter B. Cannon as the flight-or-fight response. Cannon showed that stimulation of a region of the hypothalamus leads to a series of physiological changes resulting in a 300 to 400 percent increase in blood flowing to the muscles. But it made no sense to Benson to say that TM was the *only* way to bring about this profound antistress response. So he and his colleagues dissected the TM instructions into two basic components:

1. The repetition of a word, sound, prayer, or muscular activity
2. The passive disregard of everyday thoughts when they come to mind

By examining the religious and secular literatures of the world, Benson found that the same steps existed in virtually every culture.

The earliest examples come from the Hindu Scriptures—the Upanishads—dating back to the seventh and eighth centuries B.C. It was written that to achieve a union with God, one should sit quietly, pay attention to one's breathing, and on each out-breath, repeat a word or phrase from the Scriptures, the Vedas, or the Bhagavad-Gita. When other thoughts came to mind, one should passively disregard them and come back to the repetition.

The next examples come from Judaism, dating back to the Second Temple, which is roughly from the second century B.C. to the first century A.D. In a particular school of thought, people were told to squat in a fetal-like posture, pay attention to their breathing, and on each out-breath, repeat over and over again the name of the magic seal. When other thoughts came to mind, they were to passively disregard them and come back to the repetition.

Regarding early, middle, and late Christianity, one can trace the evolution of meditative techniques through prayers dating back to the time of Christ. These were practiced by the Desert Fathers—fourth-century Christian monks who lived as hermits in the most remote part of the Egyptian desert—and ultimately codified in the fourteenth century on Mount Althos in Greece. To this day, there are hallowed Greek Byzantine monasteries espousing that people twice daily kneel quietly by themselves, pay attention to their breathing, and on each out-breath, say quietly to themselves, "Lord Jesus, have mercy" or "Lord Jesus, have mercy on us sinners." When other thoughts come to mind, the meditator is to passively disregard them and come back to the repetition.

The method of this whole process is called Hesychasm, traced back to Hesychius of Jerusalem, a fifth-century teacher of the uses of the Jesus prayer. According to Daniel Goleman, Hesychius describes prayer as "a spiritual art that releases one completely from passionate thoughts, words and evil deeds, and gives a 'sure knowledge of God the Incomprehensible.'" Hesychius describes thoughts as "enemies who are bodiless and invisible, malicious and clever and harming us, skillful, nimble and practiced in warfare," who enter through the five senses. A mind that is preoccupied with the senses or thought is distant from Jesus; one can be with him only by overcoming the lure of sensations and by attaining a silent mind. Followers are instructed to find a teacher who bares the spirit within him or her and to devote themselves to the master, obeying all commands.

Virtually the same instructions were given in fourteenth-century Judaism, where the mystical Kabbalistic tradition was evolving. Rabbi Abraham Abulafia, in one of the most detailed elaborations of Kabbalistic meditation, described a safe approach to the inner paradise:

> According to Kabbalist lore, the entry into the inner Paradise by one who has not properly prepared a foundation through self-purification can be dangerous. The Talmud tells the story of four rabbis who entered Paradise: one went mad, one died, and another lost faith; only one, Rabbi Akiba, came back in peace.

Abulafia's method calls for paying attention to one's breathing and, on each out breath, repeating the components that make up God's name, Adonois. When thoughts come to mind, they should be passively disregarded, returning to the aforementioned repetition. A similar pathway is described in Sufism, where the way to purity is the constant remembrance of God. The main mediation among Sufis is Zikr, which means "remembrance"—*La ilaha illa' llah:* "There is no god but God." According to the prophet Muhammad, "There is a polish for everything that taketh away rust; and the polish of the Heart is the invocation of Allah." Remarkably parallel traditions are found in Zen Buddhism, Shintoism, Taoism, and Confucianism—only the words are different. In the so-called primitive or shamanistic religions, people achieve similar states by chanting in time to the stamping of feet or the beating of drums—an echo of their heartbeats.

Interestingly, the same kinds of instructions are found in secular techniques, wherein relaxation or peace of mind are promoted independent of spiritual or religious ideology—for example, autogenic training, progressive relaxation, and hypnotic suggestion. (See Table 4.1.) In each case, there is an instruction to repetitiously focus on something outside the realm of ordinary thought, with passive disregard for intruding ideas or stimuli.

So, for the past twenty-five years, Benson and his colleagues have successively applied the "Relaxation Response," which embodies the fundamental components of traditional and secular techniques for achieving peace of mind. The technique has been used to diminish the complications of a range of psychophysical disorders that are thought to either be caused by or made worse by stress. It has been found useful, along with medicine, in the treatment of hypertension. Benson found, for example, that in a sample of a hundred patients, roughly 90 percent were able to maintain a lower blood pressure after being trained to elicit the Relaxation Response in a program of ten sessions spread out over a six-month period. After a three-year follow-up period, not only did blood pressures remain lower, but patients required less medication, with approximately 20 percent giving up their medications completely. Readers are cautioned that relaxation techniques for hypertension should be used only under the care and supervision of a physician, because for obvious reasons, neither overtreatment nor undertreatment is desirable.

An important benefit relative to life experience is that immediately after one elicits the Relaxation Response, the mind is more open. There appears to be enhanced communication between the right and left hemispheres of the brain. Athletes regularly elicit the Relaxation Response and then visualize their perfect event. Exceptional performance becomes a matter of simply playing out the visualization. To ensure better test results, many private schools train their students to elicit the Relaxation Response before classes and exams. With their anxiety quieted, the mind is more open and more readily receives the intended message.

Benson has shown that the Relaxation Response can be viewed as an extraordinary tool for behavior change that can be used in any desired fashion. The method of elicitation, however, is critical. Practitioners select a personally meaningful word, sound, prayer, phrase, or muscular activity for repetition. When given a choice, most people will prefer prayer (e.g., the twenty-third Psalm, Lord's Prayer, Hail Mary, or repetition of the Hebrew word for peace, "shalom." Regular practitioners often report they have made contact with their Higher Power through this process. In effect, the Relaxation Response is a tailor-made method for complementing each individual's belief system.

As a matter of fact, many patients say to me, "Thank you, doctor, for telling me to pray again. It's something that I've always wanted to do, but felt funny about. But now that you as a doctor tell me about it, it's something that I'll do." You can then utilize that mind-opening effect brought about by the elicitation of the Relaxation Response to change behavior. If you wish the person to be more positive, simply have that individual read affirmations afterwards. It can be anything from Norman Vincent Peale to Robert Schuller, to statements of truth. If the person desires better health, have them think healthy thoughts about themselves. And this isn't just a thought, but these thoughts translate, insofar as mind can affect body, into physiologic change. This is what has been proposed, for example, by the Symingtons as a way of treating cancer. They first elicit the Relaxation Response through meditation, and then they visualize white cells in Pac-man fashion sort of chewing up cancer cells. Does that work? We don't know, but it is the same basic mind/body technology that they are utilizing.

In *Your Maximum Mind*, Benson proposes a series of steps for increasing calm and optimizing life experiences. The steps can be used to promote the development of an array of artistic and recreational skills consistent with one's sense of purpose and meaning. Readers are encouraged to explore how the Relaxation Response can serve as a physiological bridge to natural highs. By participating in these steps (Table 5.5), readers will not only develop a greater sense of inner peace, but also experience enhanced feelings of pleasure, because they are more attuned to dormant proclivities, interests, and abilities that may have been suppressed by anxiety or stress.

Knowing Your Mind

Benson's meditative pathway increases calm by directing awareness to personal symbols that represent harmony and well-being. We shall now consider the alternative pathway to peace of mind, insight meditation. In *The Experience of Insight*, Joseph Goldstein developed a commonsense rationale for the Buddhist approach to meditation and offered specific instructions for practice.

According to Buddhist tradition, which has evolved since approx-

TABLE 5.5

Your Maximum Mind: A Physiological Bridge to Natural Highs

Step 1 Pick a focus word or phrase that is consistent with your philosophy of life and basic system of beliefs and values, e.g., a Christian person might choose, "The Lord is my shepherd." A non-religious person might choose "peace and harmony"; some find the word "om" to be a pleasant and spiritually inspiring sound.

Step 2 After learning to relax your muscles and attain a comfortable posture, breathe slowly and naturally, and repeat your focus word or phrase as you exhale.

Step 3 Assume a positive attitude. Deal with intruding or potentially disturbing thoughts by silently saying "so what" or "oh well," then gently return to repetition of the meaningful construct.

Step 4 Practice the technique for ten to twenty minutes once or twice daily.

Step 5 Begin to focus your thinking and behavior on pleasurable activities that are deficient in your experience.

---

imately 500 B.C., the main purpose of meditation is to come to a deeper understanding of the nature of the mind—meaning all aspects of consciousness, including intellect and feelings. In 1974, the late Tibetan teacher Chogyam Trungpa predicted that "Buddhism will come to the West as a psychology." And indeed it has.

When we consider the nature of our experience, it is clear that everything we do—whether work, family, relationships, or creativity—has some mental representation. Since much, if not all, human endeavor has its origins in our thoughts and feelings, then it would seem exceedingly worthwhile to understand the nature of our mind. The commitment to comprehend more about our own mental processes is at the core of Buddhist meditation.

One of the most obvious facts about the human psyche is that it is not static or fixed. Rather, our ideas, feelings, and fantasies are in a continuous state of evolution and flux. Also, our perceptions—the interpretations we assign to the objects and events in our midst—are colored by emotions. When we feel anger, our consciousness or awareness is tainted by hostility. When we feel love or compassion, there is increased likelihood of benevolence toward others and a positive explanation concerning events in our lives. Meditation aims to clarify the mental conditions that are associated with increased tightness, suffering, or pain, versus the qualities that lead to greater openness, ease, and well-being. But how should one choose from the array of meditative traditions and practices that are offered (e.g., Benson's Relaxation Response vs. Goldstein's insight meditation)?

An ancient Persian story helps to resolve this dilemma. The Mullah Nasrudin is a mythical Sufi teaching figure about whom there are hundreds of legends. Nasrudin is half crazy, half saint, half wise man, half fool. One day, a friend came to borrow a donkey and Nasrudin said, "I'm sorry, the donkey isn't here; I don't have it; I can't lend it to you." Just at that moment, when Nasrudin was speaking about not having the donkey, the donkey, which was outside the window, began to bray. The friend became increasingly angry and said, "How can you tell me you don't have the donkey? I hear it outside the window!" And Nasrudin, in turn, became very offended and said, "Well, who are you going to believe—me or the donkey?"

Buddha gave a very definitive answer to this question. "Don't believe anybody," he said. "Don't believe the books or the teachers and don't believe me." He advocated looking into our own mind and investigating the factors that seem conducive to greed, hatred, and delusion. These things are to be abandoned. Buddha taught that we should attend to and develop whatever actions of mind, body, and speech cultivate greater understanding and compassion. Thus, according to Joseph Goldstein, the practice of insight meditation is a matter of taking on personal responsibility for understanding the basis or purpose of our actions—for having insight. It has little or nothing to do with dogma, ritual, or religious conviction.

As a prerequisite for gaining insight—deeper understanding and sense of purpose, one should cultivate "mindfulness"—the skill of being able to attend to what is happening in each moment. Although the directive seems quite simple—to pay attention to what is happening in each instant (like now)—it's actually quite difficult to do. A cornerstone of Buddhist teaching is the delineation of succinct practice techniques to develop the quality of awareness. Practitioners are instructed to begin with the most tangible way of cultivating a strong, well-focused attention: "Be mindful of the body." What aspect of ourselves could be more accessible than paying attention to the sensations that emanate from our own physical processes, particularly the act of breathing?

Concentration on breathing develops the skill to recognize when the mind is wandering or going off, that is, losing the quality of attentiveness. It also promotes a sense of relaxation. As described earlier in the discussion of Benson's Relaxation Response, Buddhist meditators also report increased calm and feelings of well-being. As a matter of fact, breathing awareness is also introduced as a means for stress reduction or relaxation, quite apart from any meditative practice. Yet whether the technique is introduced by a mental health counselor, medical adviser, or spiritual leader, the benefits of observing our breathing while detaching ourselves from everyday thoughts are quite similar.

Beginning meditators may, however, quickly lose interest in *just* attending to routine activities such as breathing. When we consider the consequences of not being able to breathe—someone holding your head under water, for example—breathing quickly becomes our number one priority. Practitioners are reminded that in a very literal way, every breath we take is vital to sustaining our life. Not all environmentalists may be Buddhists, but Buddha would have had no objections to their campaigns for clean air.

Another aspect of mindfulness of the body is paying attention to every little thing we do: standing up, sitting down, making tea, opening the door, working at our job. A tremendous conservation of energy occurs when we develop the skill to bring our attention back to the simple movements we make throughout the day. How often do we become needlessly lost in thinking, fantasizing, or planning about some event that never takes place? As Mark Twain quipped, "I've had a lot of problems in my life, but most of them never happened." Much of our worrisome rumination is not useful—the mind, by habit, just seems to go on and on. By coming back to the simple movements of the body, we can resume concentration on the moment.

Joseph Goldstein recounts a Zen story that illustrates this point:

It seems this one person had been practicing meditation for a very long time, and he had some great insight. He was sitting in meditation and this cosmic insight unfolded, and he thought he understood the truth of things. Very excited, he went running up to his teacher, who lived in another hut in the forest. And it was raining out. Before he went in to visit his teacher, he left his shoes and umbrella outside. He went in and he bowed down to his teacher, all excited about his insight. And his Zen master simply asked him, "On which side of your shoes did you leave your umbrella?" He couldn't remember. And the Master sent him back for ten more years of practice.

The first half of meditation practice is learning to be aware. Few of us have the opportunity to devote our lives to pure meditation. How can we Westerners daily incorporate meditation into our busy lives? We have to commit to applying the practice to our everyday activities—by noting on which side of our shoes we left our umbrella. One important benefit of increasing mindfulness of our bodies, particularly while sitting, is that we become keenly aware of the tension we carry. We usually remain unaware of this stress and therefore don't release it. By increasing the awareness of our breathing, we take greater notice of the body's condition. When we become aware of the tension, rather than fighting it, we begin to release it. We let go, and stress-related illness begins to reverse its course. According to Goldstein, "There are thousands of stories from meditation centers in Thailand and Burma of very deep-seated organic diseases actually being cured through the practice. It's not the point of the practice; it's not the purpose of it; it's a byproduct."

Perception of one's mind—thoughts, emotions, feelings—is also increased. While the brain is constantly engaged in thinking—judging, remembering, planning, evaluating, processing sensory input—we spend very little time cognizant of our thoughts; that is, we leave our brain on "automatic pilot." Like a high-flying kite, our mind is often carried astray by random gusts of thought. How often in a day are we distracted by a thought and get lost in a daydream? Many times these so-called stray thoughts are a learned pattern or reaction to past experiences and cause us to react reflexively, not purposefully. How often do we get carried away by thoughts about our mother, father, lover, or children that have absolutely no basis in reality? The thought of your mother is not your mother.

Meditation allows us to explore the nature of thought and how it drives us. By increasing awareness of our thoughts, we can more easily recognize the motivation for the thought, and we can choose to act—rather than react—accordingly. Similarly, we can become more attuned to our emotions. As with thought, it is possible to observe emotions as they arise. We become more accepting and experience them on a more cognitive plane. Because we are able to filter out the "white noise" of our emotions, we can bring about increased personal calm and balance behavior, thoughts, and feelings.

The second half of meditative practice is observing the nature of all these insights, emotions, thoughts, and breaths. The one constant that binds all of these elements together is change. Life is not static or fixed, and neither are we. The greater our understanding of the nature of change, the greater our ability to let go and adapt. One of Buddha's teachings is that we cause suffering in our lives when there's attachment in the mind, because all things change. Buddhists teach their children, before they even enter grade school, that all people at some time must get old, get sick, and die.

A familiar metaphor for teaching the value of detachment describes a monkey trap widely used in Asia. A hollowed-out coconut with a small hole in the bottom is attached to a tree. A sweet is placed inside the coconut. A monkey comes along, slips its hand in, and grasps the sweet. The hole is big enough for the monkey to slip its hand in when the monkey's hand is open, but not large enough to allow the monkey to withdraw its hand when the hand is closed. Thus, the monkey is ensnared by its own greed and attachment. It is an extremely rare monkey that will open its hand, release the sweet, and thus extricate itself.

We humans place ourselves in the same predicament. We are trapped by our own attachments. We refuse to acknowledge that we are the cause of our suffering, and we place the blame on external causes. It takes a great deal of sensitivity and openness to accept our responsibility and learn how to release it. When we are successful, our bodies, minds, and lives become more harmonious and free. Goldstein provides the instructions, shown in Table 5.6, for insight meditation.

The Creative Response

The gift of creativity allows for an infinite variety of novel solutions to a staple host of ancient problems. The unique patterns we develop in the triad of human endeavor—work, love, and play—illuminate meaning and purpose against T. S. Eliot's rude backdrop of "birth and copulation and death—those are all the facts when you come down to brass tacks." Yet personal talent and ingenuity are insufficient, in and of themselves, to provide pleasure and meaning

TABLE 5.6
Goldstein's Instructions for Insight Meditation

- Sit fairly still and stable. Frequent changes of position break the concentration. If you become very uncomfortable and painful, shift, but for the most part try to sit as still as possible. Arrange your hands in any comfortable position, either on your knees or in your lap.
- Let your eyes close gently and softly. Take a few deep breaths to connect yourself with the breathing. Begin to feel the rise and fall of the abdomen that happens with each breath. When you breathe in, there's a rising moving of the abdomen, an expansion. When you breathe out there's a natural falling or contraction. Focus your awareness on that movement, feeling the sensations of the rising movement, and the falling movement. Be aware of the movement—from the very beginning, to the middle, and end of the falling movement.
- Don't rush or force the breathing in any way. Let the rising and falling happen in its own time. See how subtle and careful your awareness and attention can be.
- Make a soft mental note of rising at the beginning of the rising movement, and a soft mental note of falling at the beginning of the falling movement. Just a soft whisper in the mind. The word "rising" . . . "falling." . . .
- If sounds become distracting and call your attention away from the rising and falling, make a note of hearing, focusing your attention just on the vibration of the sound. Make the note "hearing," "hearing," without thinking of the cause of the sounds, just experiencing the actual phenomenon of hearing, and then return again to the rising and falling.
- Let the sounds simply arise and pass away, noting "hearing" when they are distracting and calling your attention, and returning in a very careful and subtle way to rising and falling of the abdomen.
- If any sensations in the body become predominant—tightness, pressure, aching, vibration, tingling, itching—make a note of the particular sensation observing it carefully. Observe what happens to it as you notice. Does it get stronger? Does it get weaker? Does it disappear?
- And again return to the rising and falling. See how carefully you can feel each breath, making the soft note of "rise" and "fall," and if sounds distract you, calling your attention away, make a note of "hearing." And return to the rising and falling.
- If there are any strong sensations in the body that are more predominant than the breath, make a note of the sensation, feeling it, observing it, and noticing what happens as you note it. Does it get stronger? Does it get weaker? How does it change? And return to the rising and falling.
- Whenever you become aware of a thought in the mind, make a note of "thinking," trying to notice as close to the beginning as possible. Observe what happens to the thought as you note it. Does it continue? Does it disappear?

TABLE 5.6
(continued)

- Keep the mind alert and wakeful, noting in each moment the rise and fall of the breath, or hearing, or sensations in the body, or thinking—aware in each moment of the predominant object.
- See how carefully you can feel each breath: the entire movement of the rising, the entire movement of the falling.
- As soon as you are aware that the mind is wandering, make a note of "thinking," observe what happens to the thought as you note it, come back to the breathing.
- And if there is any strong mind state or emotion: of boredom, of interest, happiness, sadness, anger, fear, compassion—if any strong emotion should arise, that also should be noted. Feel it, be aware of it, and return again to the breath.
- Feel each rising and falling carefully and accurately, making the soft mental note.
- Make a note of any strong, predominant sensation in the body that may call your attention away from the breathing.
- If there are any images or pictures in the mind, make a note of "seeing"; observe what happens to the picture or image as you note it; then return to the rise and fall.
- Keep your attention on the breath, on any sounds which may become predominant, or any sensations, noting also images as they may come to mind, keeping the mind wakeful and alert in each moment, seeing all phenomena arising and passing away.

---

throughout the lifespan. In the end, extended pleasure derives from finding a confluence between biochemical titillation and uplifting human values.

In *The Farther Reaches of Human Nature,* Abraham Maslow writes, "The concept of creativeness and the concept of the healthy self-actualizing, fully human person seem to be coming closer and closer together, and may perhaps turn out to be the same thing." The creative response is the natural result of integrating the inner resources we have described thus far: optimism, guiding principles, pleasurable activities, and personal calm.

The kernel of creativity appears during infancy—the impulse to discover new sensations and how things work, the drive to experiment with different methods of thinking, feeling, and behaving. Indeed, according to Walt Whitman, childhood bursts with creative adventure:

There was a child went forth every day,
And the first object he look'd upon, that object he became,
And that object became part of him for the day, or a certain part of
    the day,
Or for many years or stretching cycles of years.
The early lilacs became part of this child,
And grass and white and red morning-glories, and red and white
    cloves and the song of the phoebe bird,
And the third-month lambs and the sow's pink-faint litter, and the
    mare's foal and the cow's calf,
And the noisy brood of the barnyard or by the mire of the pond-side,
And the fish suspending themselves so curiously below there, and the
    beautiful curious liquid,
And the water plants with their graceful flat heads, all became part of
    him.

Discovery—whether seeing a oneness between all forms of matter, manifesting latent talents or skills, finding beauty through harmony and wholeness, or uncovering some mystery of cause and effect—opens the channels of primary bliss. And the roots of discovery emerge during childhood, when spontaneity flourishes and self-consciousness is yet unknown. In Asia, the image of water is frequently used as a metaphor for the spirit of creativity. Water is entirely responsive to the elements it touches. When flowing through canyons, it becomes a river; when blocked by a cavern, it journeys around; but when you submerge a pail beneath its surface, immediately and perfectly it conforms to the pail's contours. Water is like the mind of a child—receptive to circumstance. According to Kenneth Kraft, Buddhist scholar at Lehigh University, "A person who is deeply responsive to the conditions in which he finds himself will be creative."

When we take note of the thought processes of self-actualized people, we find obvious links to childhood wonders. Einstein queried about what it would be like to ride on a beam of light; Picasso mused, Howard Gardner tells us, over what would happen if we fragmented objects and painted them in their component parts.

Picasso at twenty could paint as well as anyone in the world; Einstein at twenty could do physics as well as anyone in the world. . . . They captured something about what it was like to be a child, both in the sense of being a free explorer of a domain, somebody with the whole world open to them, but also puzzling about the sort of things children puzzle about.

But for most, the naïveté and responsiveness of childhood become lost in the sociohormonal deluge of adolescence, en route to becoming an adult. The disappearance of a playful child is an image that arises in the Greek myth of Demeter and Persephone. Clarissa Pinkola Estes, noted Jungian scholar, views the story as a metaphor for the creative process. By analyzing the components of the tale, we can better understand the ebb and flow of our own creative energies, thereby enhancing the possibility of self-actualization.

> Demeter is a symbol of maternal beauty in Greek mythology. The Earth exists in an idyllic state because of Demeter's fertility and potential for future children. Persephone, her playful teenage daughter, is a source or great pride to her mother. The youthful Persephone finds her contribution to earthly splendor is aimless play.

The undirectedness of Persephone's actions are essential to the creative process. Henri Poincare, the ninteenth-century mathematician, proposed that the first step to inventiveness is in the ability to immerse oneself in a problem—uncritically seeking any information that might be relevant. According to Estes, aimlessness is vital because the creative mind is neither rational nor focused; it is more likely to be imbued with sensations or feeling states that allow people to create from their soul rather than from a place of logic and reason.

> The Earth cracked open and Hades, the god of the Underworld, sped by in his chariot, abducting Persephone and carrying her back to his place of darkness.

The inevitable recession of spontaneity is a source of alarm for many who embark on the creative journey. Estes explains that "something from the unconscious has come and snatched away that playfulness, that lack of direction and meandering that leads to their creative spirit." Poincare describes this phase of the creative process as incubation, wherein much of what occurs is outside the mind's awareness. The unconscious, which is rich in imagery and feelings, is in many ways more intellectually adept than the conscious mind.

Actually, we are more open to insights from this aspect of our being in moments of reverie—when we are not actively trying to do or think about anything. Nolan Bushnell, who founded the Atari Company, became inspired to develop a prolific videogame while flicking sand on the beach.

In the myth, Demeter becomes aware of Persephone's absence and becomes so disturbed that she loses her fertility. All the crops die and Earth becomes a horrible, barren place. Demeter, devoid of passion and power, wanders about listlessly in search of her lost daughter.

The message of this component of the story is quite clear. As Daniel Goleman writes in *The Creative Spirit,* "When the darkness is seen as a necessary prelude to the creative light, one is less likely to ascribe frustration to personal inadequacy or label it 'bad.'" When the inescapable impasse presents itself along the path of a creative project—when things come to an apparent standstill—one should avoid the pitfalls of self-doubt and anxiety and instead begin the search for hidden material. Estes views the seizure of Persephone as a kind of creative death wish, something that hopes for or wishes for death or that, like the Phoenix, can rise again and grow in a new direction.

In the myth, Baubo, a female goddess of obscenity, comes to Demeter, who is by now haggard and fatigued. Baubo presents a lewd dance and begins telling obscene jokes which cause Demeter to break into laughter. As a result of this humor, Demeter regains her direction and her thinking becomes lucid.

To be sure, humor lubricates the wheels of creativity. When you take time out to laugh at the absurdity of a situation, suddenly you become free to sift information from apparent irrelevancies. In fact, as Aubrey Bauch once said, "Creativity is the ability to see the relativity of the absurd."

The medicine woman Hecate—the one who interprets between the land of the living and the land of the dead—queries, "Who do you think took your daughter?" This constitutes a breakthrough for Demeter who never considered that another being might be involved in Demeter's disappearance. They decide to ask Helios, the Sun, to reveal what happened because Helios sees all. Helios reveals that "Hades took your daughter, I saw it, I saw it all."

Poincare identified this state in the creative process as illumination; suddenly, the answer appears as if from nowhere. There is a feeling of jubilation, a sense of "Eureka! I found it!" or "This is it!"

When Demeter finally gets the answer to who took her daughter, her trial is by no means complete. She must now enter what Poincare described as the final stage of creativity: translation. Converting your idea into an actual product (an invention, a painting, an essay, or a book—something that is useful to others)—this is the finale of the creativity process and usually the stage of greatest tribulation. As Thomas Edison is credited with saying, "Ninety-nine percent of genius is perspiration—not inspiration—sticking to it is the genius."

> Demeter now has to figure out how to get her daughter back. As things go, the people of Greece become involved. They appeal to Zeus—most powerful of all the gods—to restore Persephone to Demeter because the barren land is causing the people to die.

Ultimately, the creative process involves the inclusion of others. In fact, creativity does not reside entirely within the individual; it is a social phenomenon, rather than purely psychological. Creativity, according to Dean Simington, occurs when three basic elements coincide: novelty, appropriateness in audience, and reception to its impact.

> According to the myth, Zeus, who had conspired with Hades, giving him his blessing to steal Persephone, must now reconsider his deal because of the extent of suffering that has been created. He decides to reverse his decision and tells Hades to restore Persephone. Hades, who has already made the young beauty his bride and queen, refutes the injunction by professing his love for her. Zeus then strikes the deal that if Persephone hasn't eaten anything in the Underworld she can be restored unequivocally. If, on the other hand, she has tasted something, then she'll have to remain in the Underworld part of the time. Hades, in a fit of desperation, stuffs a pomegranate in Persephone's mouth. She tries to spit it out, but accidentally swallows six seeds. As a result, Zeus decides that Persephone can live with her mother six months of the year and with Hades during the other six.

While the myth of Demeter and Persephone is used to explain seasonal changes, it also illuminates the fact that creativity is cyclic. It is not utopic and uninterrupted; creatvity must be lost and restored in order to assess its true value and meaning. Estes likens Hades to what may be termed the editor, director, or critic—that part of us which judges our efforts and ourselves as unworthy. Goleman identifies the following "creativity killers" frequently inflicted on children: surveillance, evaluation, excessive rewards, competition, overcontrol, choice restriction, pressure, and—the biggest assassin—structured, limited time.

Estes believes that many of the harsh punishments we inflict on ourselves and our children stem from complexes—a set of emotions with their own agenda: "If you understand the negative father and negative mother complex, you get a better idea of exactly what is stealing your creativity away from you. . . . The editor can be exceptionally cruel and debilitating. There is no other thing that makes creativity go away [faster] than that cold killing force in the psyche that tells you that you and your work are inadequate. . . . There is a part of the psyche that bleeds when it hears those things and there's a blood loss to the [creative] energy."

We can't prevent Persephone from being stolen from us. When our creativity takes a sabbatical, laughter, twilight imagery, meditation, and dream journaling can locate our Persephone, negotiate with our Zeus, and restrict the pull of Hades.

Orchestrating Fitness

Bring the body; the mind will follow.
> —*Alcoholics Anonymous aphorism,*
> *author unknown*

There I was, 6 AM, standing in the middle of the room looking like Don King on a bad hair day. I had the coloring of an albino male. I felt breaded and fried, shaked and baked, a crustacean in a unitard. I was surrounded by hundreds of me, thousands of me, mirrors everywhere. It was horrifying . . .

Aerobics—there, I've admitted it. There's nothing worse than spending an hour with women who would have their taste buds waxed if bumpy tongues went out-of-style—Spandex before breakfast, lipo before lunch. And there they were, surrounding me, parading around in, "bouffy" hair, looking like cotton candy live. . . .

I spend a lot of time alternating between hating the people that join clubs and joining clubs and hating myself.

> —*Gwen Macsai, on National Public Radio's "Morning Edition"*

Probably nothing captures the essence of optimal living more than the word *happiness. Webster's* dictionary gives many definitions for *happiness,* most of which fail to convey the emotional experience of a truly happy life. This is not surprising: good feelings and positive emotions are the result of enhanced neurotransmission in the Reward Center located in the limbic system, while words are human constructions designed to articulate these feelings. It is no wonder happiness is hard to describe. It has a subjective nature, and so we recognize it when we experience it. It is also true that a happy life is a healthy life. Many scientists believe that old-fashioned joy, whether exhibited by optimism, curiosity, or just serenading the sweetness of spring, not only makes life worth living but makes it last longer. Euphoria seems to protect us from the stressful assaults of living at the turn of the twenieth century. Joyful people are known to outlive their negative, whining contemporaries.

During a short visit to China, one of us (Sunderwirth) found that the Chinese exhibit a philosophy that well summarizes optimal living; every toast to the foreigner, as well as to fellow Chinese, is preceded by the phrase "Good fortune, long life, happiness." While good fortune may be elusive, clearly, long life without happiness is not a desirable goal. One of the best ways to ensure long life and happiness is through creating and maintaining excellent health.

The same author also spent considerable time in Mexico and South America. In South America, optimal living is characterized by the standard toast *"Amor, dinero, y salud"* ("Love, money, and health"). He was often asked by his South American hosts which of the three he thought was most important. His answer? Health. His hosts agreed, for without health, money and love cannot be fully appreciated.

There is also an Arab proverb stressing the role of health in a full and rewarding life:

He who has health has hope.
And he who has hope has everything.

For example, when Alfred, a health-conscious yet poorly paid church pastor in his fifties, went for his yearly physical, the doctor, a wealthy physician with a respected practice, told him, following the exam, "I'd give up my practice for your health." But we don't have to give up our income, family, or friends to obtain and maintain good health; we don't have to compromise one for the other.

So it seems that even cross-culturally, the wisdom of the ages appreciates that optimal living involves a long and happy life, characterized by a healthy body, a sound mind full of hope, loving relationships and a comfortable standard of living.

According to David Meyers, author of *The Pursuit of Happiness: Who Is Happy—and Why*, research indicates that some of the activities, behaviors, and attitudes that support happiness and satisfaction are these:

1. Aerobically fit and healthy bodies
2. Realistic goals and expectations
3. Supportive friendships
4. An intimate, sexually warm marriage (the Chinese symbol for "good" is a man and woman together)
5. A faith that provides support, purpose, and acceptance

It is no coincidence that the first requisite is a fit and healthy body. Other experts have noted this. Diane Swanbrow lists several steps to happiness, including the following:

Energize yourself: Run, play a sport, dance—the choice is yours, as long as you keep aerobically fit. Whether the feeling of well-being produced by exercise is due to the release of endorphins—the brain's natural painkillers—or something else, researchers agree that fitness is one reliable road to happiness.

In this chapter, we concentrate on achieving and maintaining physical as well as mental health. Actually, the two cannot be separated completely, since the master control center for both mental and physical well-being is the brain: what affects one affects the other. As we shall see later, a prime example of this interplay of mind and body is the manner in which one's mental attitude affects his or her physical health.

The Constitution of the United States guarantees us "the pursuit of happiness: but not happiness itself. This we must achieve to a large degree by our own efforts. Unfortunately, many people do not know how to go about achieving happiness. Even more distressing is that some people believe that happiness, fun, pleasure, and interest in the body are somehow too hedonistic and even sinful. The concept that any pleasure derived from our bodies is sinful has a long history in religious circles. St. Thomas Aquinas described the prevalent religious thinking of his day concerning marital sex, the most intense emotional and pleasurable experience the combination of body and mind can generate:

Some say that when pleasure is the chief motive of the marriage act it is a mortal sin; that when it is an indirect motive it is a venial sin; and that when it spurns the pleasure altogether, and is displeasing, it is

wholly void of venial sin so that it would be a mortal sin to take pleasure when it is offered, but that perfection requires one to detest it.

Although St. Thomas Aquinas did not completely concur with
this belief, he reluctantly admitted that "neither will it be always a
mortal sin to seek pleasure therein."

Fortunately, the mainstream of religious and secular thinking has
moved away from the belief that pleasure associated with our bodies
is, if not sinful, at least frivolous and unessential to our lives. It is
now becoming more obvious that taking pleasure in our bodies is a
crucial component of not only a happy but also a healthy life. A
basic premise of optimal living is that satisfaction with our bodies
contributes importantly to mental health and happiness.

Unfortunately, an active interest in maintaining a healthy body
can be a two-edged sword. The synergism of mind and body can
turn against us if we allow virulent thoughts to pollute our body
image. The present svelte-crazed desire to look like Cher or Bruce
Lee has caused many people with perfectly healthy physiques to
abhor their bodies and subsequently themselves.

If we are to achieve the life to which we are all entitled, we must
learn how to use our brain to rid ourselves of any lingering toxic
thoughts about our bodies that creep into our minds. Only then can
we use these same mental techniques to move on to those heights of
pleasure and joy which we associate with total wellness.

Many of these negative thoughts about ourselves in general and
our bodies in particular are faulty perceptions created by others,
often accidentally. Consider an incident in the life of Sheila, a Midwestern housewife in her forties who has battled anorexia for most
of her life.

> What got me into anorexic behavior was my grandfather. On this par-
> ticular Sunday, there were thirty of my male relatives sitting around.
> We were eating dinner. I walked through with a plate of food, and my
> grandfather, who was kind of a jokester, said in front of thirty men,
> "Here comes my only fat granddaughter."

That single, unintentionally harmful, offhanded remark by someone she dearly loved started Sheila on a lifelong battle in which food
became an all-consuming preoccupation.

Thinking of Your Body

Let's consider another real-life example of body image gone awry. Andrea recoils in horror as she steps on the scale and reads the tell-tale numbers, reminding her that she has gained almost 2 pounds since she last weighed herself. She is now up to 119 pounds, 4 pounds over her normal 115 pounds, the same she weighed as a high school cheerleader in 1963. The fact that her friends think she's a marvelous physical specimen seems to make no difference to her. She is in excellent health, has boundless energy, and rarely gets sick. In her leisuretime she may hike fifteen miles in a day or ride a bicycle thirty-five miles. In her profession, she often works up to ten to twelve hours a day, five days a week. Yet when she looks in the mirror, instead of seeing the perfectly normal, shapely body that she has, she sees the slight rise around her midriff. This appears in her mind like an inflated inner tube from a Mack truck, and her hips and thighs as something that would be more fitting for an elephant. She goes into a momentary depression, her self-esteem falling to the floor as her imagination catapults the entirely normal figure in the mirror to something that, in her mind, resembles Fat Albert, the character made famous by Bill Cosby. Andrea promises to punish herself for this weight gain. She vows not to eat breakfast (the worst possible thing she could do); to eat only an apple for lunch, cottage cheese and a salad for dinner; and to take a brisk, three-mile walk before bedtime. Of course, this unrealistic and unhealthy promise is broken, as she is so hungry at bedtime that she is unable to sleep. She gets up around 11:00 P.M., craving food, especially carbohydrates. Biochemically, her brain, through a serotonin feedback mechanism, recognizes the dangerously low level of carbohydrates and literally commands her to eat them.

Andrea has unknowingly set herself up to fail; skipping breakfast is a sure way to bring on an eating binge later in the day. Further, exercising before going to bed, especially vigorously exercising following carbohydrate deprivation, not only is neurochemically foolish if one wishes to sleep, but also can be physically dangerous. Too often we, like Andrea, are unable to be content or find pathways to pleasure if we feel we are grossly overweight—even if we are not. Unfortunately, it is true that our perception may become our reality.

Our brain, which can be our ally, can also become our worst enemy as we allow adverse thoughts about our body to infect our mind.

A prerequisite to optimal living is a positive image of ourselves and our bodies.

Morton Harmatz of the University of Massachusetts wrote, "You are as fat as you think." This belief was based on his research, in which he found that many normal and even underweight women considered themselves too fat. Of course, these women were "fat" only when compared to beauty contest winners, who are usually 15 to 20 pounds underweight. Playboy Playmates have, on the average lost 20 pounds over the past twenty years. Being this much underweight is not especially healthy and even borders on being unhealthy. Fashion models are even at greater risk for health problems, especially eating disorders.

Andrea is divorced and at present is in a meaningful and satisfying relationship. Her children are grown and have become very successful in their chosen careers. Now, instead of enjoying her newfound freedom from home responsibility and an unhappy marriage, she has become preoccupied with her weight. For almost a year, she has been punishing herself to lose weight that she does not really need to lose.

Andrea has fallen into the diet–compulsive eating–guilt cycle discussed by Marcia Hutchinson in her book *Transforming Body Image*. People who know Andrea say, "How silly of her to make such a fuss over her perfectly normal and healthy body!" Her friends don't take her seriously, and this adds to her frustration. Unfortunately, the painful truth is that she is only one of many thousands, and perhaps millions, of women in this country with healthy body weight whose internal body image has little to do with their external physical body. Harmatz's research found that even among underweight women, 83 percent considered themselves to be of normal weight and 36 percent of normal-weight women thought they were overweight. As long as your mental image of your body is negative, no amount of shaping through either exercise or diet will satisfy you. You have to use your mind as well as your body in order to reshape your self-image.

Through either real or, in too many cases, imagined faulty bodies, far too many people in this country are, unfortunately, prevented from finding their individual road to joyful living. Regardless of whether their "faulty" bodies are real or imagined, steps can and must be taken to correct them. (Later in this chapter, we discuss ways to obtain and maintain truly healthy bodies.) These steps are different from those which should be taken by people whose need to "shape up" is mostly in their minds.

An Andrea looks in the mirror and once again sees her perfectly normal and healthy body, her mind becomes her enemy as she allows a distorted perception to invade her private world. If you hate your body, it's hard to take pleasure in anything, except possibly the temporary escape of overeating. In Andrea's case, her imagination is preventing optimal enjoyment of what could be one of the best times of her life. If left unconfronted, her imagination could escalate and prevent her from obtaining pleasure in numerous aspects of her life.

If the imagination can be powerful enough to negatively influence our self-perception, why can't it be used to repair our body image? Obviously, it can. Perhaps you think that the power of imagination is just "psychobabble," that what we really have to do is starve ourselves and exercise until we drop to obtain the body we want (but may not need). To show that this is not true, let's test the power of imagination on your emotions as well as your physical state. Suppose that you are the person who experienced the burglar attack described in Chapter 3. It is ten days after the attack, and you are calmly sitting in your office, working on some rather meaningless paperwork. As your thoughts begin to wander, they suddenly return to the attack, and you begin to relive the experience in your mind. Immediately, the locus coeruleus in your brain increases the output of norepinephrine. Norepinephrine pathways extending from the locus coeruleus into the amygdala change your tranquil emotional state into one of extreme fright. Other neuronal pathways extend from the locus coeruleus into the hypothalamus, activating the hypothalamic pituitary adrenal axis (HPA), resulting in the release of adrenaline (see Chapter 3). As adrenaline surges through your body, your heart rate accelerates, your palms begin to sweat, and your breathing becomes shallow. This neurochemical cascade produces an emotional and physical state different only by degrees from that during the initial burglary incident.

Now try hard to do the same thing yourself. Concentrating deeply, think of an extremely positive event that occurred sometime in your life, one in which you felt pure ecstasy. Block out external stimuli, and imagine that you're reliving that pleasurable event. First, get comfortable. Then concentrate: imagine the most thrilling or pleasurable event of your life, the one event in which you felt the most pride and elation. Take a full minute or two to reexperience that event. For example, image the first time you fell in love. The classic experience of new lovers, when all of life transcends normalcy and one is swept up in a world of grace and beauty, is the outcome of the chemistry of love. When love is new, people feel friendlier and are more carefree; joy is discovered in the most mundane. Everything from the weather to the food one eats takes on an almost surreal goodness. Because of this heightened sensitivity and awareness, life is transformed.

If you truly revived this episode in your mind, you'll experience sensations and emotions not unlike those experienced in the original.

Powerful mental imagery plays an important part in shaping all aspects of our lives It has been said, "If you can imagine it, you can do it." In fact, before we can do, we must imagine. This is why goal setting is so powerful. Probably nowhere is the power of imaging more dramatic than in the lives of athletes preparing for competition. Dick Fosburg, who startled the athletic world in 1968 at the Mexico City Olympics with his unorthodox high-jumping style, describes his method of success:

> I began to develop my new style during high school competition, when my body seemed to react to the challenge of the bar. I became charged by the desire and will to achieve success. Then I developed a thorough process in order to repeat a successful jump: I would "psyche" myself up; create a picture; "feel" a successful jump—the perfect jump; and develop a positive attitude to make the jump. My success came from the visualization and imaging process.

Tom Schuler, who won the U.S. Pro Championship in 1987, stresses that focus and mental preparation are even more important than rest, nutrition, and training the final week before the event.

Jackie Joyner-Kersee, probably the greatest athlete of the twentieth century, has regular "workouts" reclining in an easy chair with her eyes closed, imaging a flawless performance. Also, watch the divers at the Olympics as they stand on the end of the board, their eyes closed, as they image the intricate movements that will be required in the next few seconds. They spend at least as much time imaging their dive as is required by the dive itself.

The efficacy of imaging the successful completion of a task or performance is not a trade secret of world-class athletes. In fact, daydreaming fits into this category. An example of how a person can use this method through a more formal means than daydreaming was witnessed one day by one of us (Sunderwirth). Kathy, an executive secretary on a college campus, is known for her ability to play the trumpet in a brass quintet. One day, she was seen doing something odd. She was sitting in her office chair, her fingers flying up and down in midair. Her breath was calculated, her lips were pursed, and her feet were tapping. Kathy was playing an imaginary trumpet! When asked, Kathy explained that, before a big performance, she commonly practices in this manner, "playing" the notes and "hearing" the music. This imaging helps her sense the flow of the score, she further explained. Kathy says that this exercise of imagining greatly improves her performance. She adds that it can also be done at midnight without disturbing her sleeping children and neighbors!

How does imaging work? There are several theories, but one that seems obvious is the effect of imaging on strengthening neural pathways in the brain. As one watches an Olympic diver, it is hard not to be awed by the realization that it is the development of new neuronal pathways in the brain that is as responsible for the diver's performance as for his or her muscular development. Development of muscle tissue is meaningless to these athletes without the accompanying development of neuronal pathways that allow the muscles to perform their intricate maneuvers. The neurons of the brain have a plasticity that enables new pathways to be developed as we learn new material. Watch the diver poised at the end of the board. You can almost see these neuronal paths light up as she or he imagines the next few seconds. Since performance training is as much mental as physical, repetition of the performance in the mind strengthens the neuronal pathways in much the same way as actual performance strengthens the muscles of the body.

But most of us are not going to be concert musicians, much less Olympic divers. We would just like to feel better about our bodies and look at them with pride. We can do it!

Sheri, a returning student at a midwestern university, describes her experience in using imaging in a number of areas in her life. Let's look at how she used imagery to shape her body, both physically and mentally:

> My most recent use of imaging has been with weight loss. There was a day, about four months ago, when I stepped on the scale and it read 184 pounds. I was shocked that I had that much weight on my 5'2" body! In fact, I found it so unbelievable that I weighed myself on three other scales before I was convinced that my scale wasn't deceiving me—I was obese! That night, I started a program that has led to a loss of 30 pounds in the past four months. First, I started paying attention to the fat content of what I ate. Second, I started a regular exercise program. Third, and what I consider a vital step, I imagined myself as the thin person I want to be. I use this image on a daily basis. I visualize myself being thinner. I "feel" what it is like to be comfortable in my clothes and with my image. I imagine my metabolism increasing. I don't have a weight goal. In fact, I've only weighed myself once since I began. Now that I imagine myself to be a healthy, fit person, I don't need to worry about the weight. I am convinced that my "outside" will soon look exactly the way my mind "sees" it.

She also has used imagery to soften the shock of returning to college after sixteen years:

> The second major use of imaging in my life was when I returned to college after a sixteen-year hiatus. The anxiety I felt was almost overwhelming. After all, I had spent the last sixteen years making "hammy sandwiches," and my vocabulary had become limited to "Mommy said *No*!" I was sure my brain had become mush. I realized, however, that I could succeed if I "imagined" myself being a successful student. I visualized myself as a student for weeks before I actually became one. I would imagine myself in a classroom literally "soaking up" all of the information. Then I drew a mental image of myself taking a test and being able to recall all of that information when I needed to. I told myself over and over again that I was a great student. I am still using this image, and my 3.96 grade point average is proof that I have indeed become a successful student.

Finally, she has successfully used imaging to quit smoking:

> I first used imaging when I quit smoking eight years ago. I visualized myself not needing the cigarettes. I would remind myself of this image every time I lit up. Then one morning, I woke up and I no longer

needed the cigarettes. I was able to put them down and quit. I had become the nonsmoker I had imagined myself to be.

As important to a good body image as not being overweight is the manner in which we carry the weight we have. Even a slender body looks awful if the posture is poor (shoulders forward and bent, back curved as in a premature dowager's hump, head down and forward, stomach out, etc.). If we don't have enough respect for our bodies to show them at their best, how can be expect others to have a positive image of us? No matter what you think of your body, don't let anyone else think that you consider it less than perfect. Walk erect, back straight, gut in, head over your shoulders (not in your lap), and chest out. Walk as if you are about to attend the most important meeting of your life. Good posture in walking, standing, and sitting tells others that you are in control of your life. Walk confidently and others will think you are confident. Soon you will be confident. General Douglas MacArthur did not exactly have the body of a Greek god, but he walked ramrod-straight with a bold stride. The air of confidence he generated among those around him had nothing to do with his actual physical body. The aura he conveyed to others, and in all probability to himself as well, was one of complete control.

Unfortunately, many of us must work in environments that are unconducive to maintaining a positive attitude. But this should not deter us from projecting an attitude of confidence to those around us. We can overcome negative surroundings by projecting a positive self-image through assertive posture and perceived cheerful attitude. Dan, a college administrator, worked for several years under a tyrannical college president who took delight in humiliating those who worked under him. Everyone in the college was aware of this behavior, and many felt sympathy (something no administrator wants) for those administrators under his jurisdiction. Dan, determined not to appear browbeaten, would always leave his office where others would see him, in full stride, shoulders back, and greet everyone with a friendly "Hello" or "Good morning," even if he were about to attend a dreaded meeting with the president. His colleagues thought, "Here's one guy who knows how to handle the president."

One of the statements in the very clever *Life's Little Instruction Book*, by H. Jackson Brown, Jr., is this:

Be brave.
If you're not, act brave.
No one will know the difference.

Actually, if you act brave enough times, you will become more brave. It's all a matter of attitude and imagination. William James once said:

The greatest discovery of my generation is that a human being can alter his life by altering his attitude.

Exercise: No Pain—Much Gain

The fact that many people needlessly agonize over their body shape does not negate the hard fact that more than 34 million Americans are, in fact, overweight. There are those who really do need to lose weight, not only for cosmetic reasons but, more important, for reasons of physical health as well as mental health. As stated earlier, it is difficult to imagine a life of optimal living without optimal health, both physical and mental. Obviously, it is true that many, through no fault of their own, feel that they are destined for poor health, due to some handicap. We must remember, however, that good health is not defined as the absence of disease or handicap, anymore than poor health is necessarily defined as the presence of these afflictions. There are large numbers of people who are in poor health but have no disease or handicap. Therefore, it is vitally important that each of us make every effort to maximize our health to the limit of our physical ability. Fortunately, exercise can be a totally renewing experience, both in body and mind, even for those who have handicaps or disease. For now, let us concentrate on strengthening the body, always remembering that brain and body are not separate entities and that what strengthens one will strengthen the other.

For all of us, a strong and vital body, within the limits of our ability, should be a key milestone on the road to "good fortune, long life, and happiness." If you are serious about striving for a healthy body, there is good news. Weight reduction, accompanied by an increase in body tone and strength, is possible and within the reach of all of us by a sustained and conscientious program of exercise and proper diet. The bad news is that these are the *only* ways. Until one becomes committed to these truths, there is little hope for long-term optimal health.

More and more, people are realizing this truth and are taking steps (some good, some bad) in an attempt to achieve a stronger and more healthy body. The flooding of the market with various types of exercise equipment, as well as workout programs by celebrities, is an indication of this national concern. Unfortunately, the body shapes of these exercise gurus are virtually unattainable by all but the genetically predisposed and/or the pathologically dedicated. How many workingmen and -women can take the time out of their busy schedules to exercise several hours per day to look like Jane Fonda or Jean-Claude Van Damme? Unfortunately, the potential for disappointment when we fail to achieve these figures is enormous and is reflected in the high rate at which people discontinue their programs.

One purpose of this chapter is to lead the reader to a better understanding of the significant whole-life benefits of a sensible exercise program, not necessarily one supposedly leading to a cover model's body. As we shall see, a sensible exercise program is not just for those who wish to lose weight; it is also a prescription for all of us who wish to participate in the fullness of life. This is true for those who are not overweight as well as for those who are.

So, what is a "sensible" exercise program, for both the overweight individual and those who are not? Doesn't this word *sensible* sound a little wimpy? Isn't the old marathoner adage "No pain, no gain" the real way to exercise for good health as well as muscular fitness? Absolutely not! Health benefits are not directly proportional to the total amount of energy expended. If your exercise of choice is running and you run more than twenty miles a week, you are running for more than reasons of health. Although this level of commitment is not necessarily harmful, don't expect greater health benefits than those who run twelve to fifteen miles a week. The operative word here is *health*, not *marathonlike endurance*.

Exercise of Choice

To be effective, exercise must suit your lifestyle, including your personal and professional life. Finding a rewarding exercise that you enjoy should not be difficult, since hundreds of different options are available. All of these alternatives can be broken down into five categories: isometric, isotonic, isokinetic, anaerobic, and aerobic.

1. *Isometric exercise* (beach bully kicks sand in the face of 97-pound weakling). Charles Atlas popularized this form of exercise, which he termed "Dynamic Tension." In isometric exercise, muscles push hard against each other. While this does produce a gain in strength   (Ninety-seven-pound-weakling-turned-hero-of-the-beach punches out beach bully. "What a build! He's already famous for it!"), isometrics do not lead to overall body conditioning. The advantage of such exercises is that they can be performed anywhere, anytime. This is beneficial for those who must sit for long periods or who are immobilized. Isometrics enable such persons to obtain some muscle strength. It is believed, however, that isometrics should not be the only type of exercise performed by those individuals who have coronary heart disease. In general, isometrics do not constitute a satisfactory overall conditioning exercise. They are, though, the least expensive of the different types of exercise, since not even special shoes are required.

2. *Isotonic exercise* (pumping iron). The difference between isometric and isotonic exercise is that in isotonic exercise, the muscles contract with the accompanying movement of the joints. Weightlifting and exercises such as pushups are examples of this type of exercise. Generally speaking, weight-training programs oriented primarily toward body building are based on isotonic exercises. While weight training can be a central part of an overall exercise program, it shouldn't be considered the complete program if one's desire is to improve fitness and health. A number of popular magazines are devoted entirely to this type of exercise; *Muscle and Fitness* is one example. While pumping iron might lead to the type of physique (but God only knows why anyone would want it) shown on the covers of such magazines, it is definitely to be avoided as the sole source of exercise by individuals who have a history of heart disease. On the other hand, it is very helpful in building strength—but, again, should be accompanied by other forms of exercise.

R$_x$ for aging. It has been found that weight training can be very beneficial when combined with other forms of exercise for individuals who have adopted or been forced into a sedentary lifestyle. Recent research has shown that the introduction of programs involving moderate weight-bearing exercise has resulted in significant health benefits for seniors in convalescent homes. Among these benefits are decreased incidence of osteoporosis, increased muscle tone, improved mobility and flexibility, and, just as important, enhanced elevated mental acuity and mood. You're never too old to exercise. In another study, involving ninety-year-olds, many of whom had arthritis and coronary disease, exercising three times a week produced gains in muscle size, strength, and ambulatory ability. Greg Gutfield, writing in *Prevention* magazine, describes the research of William Evans of Tufts University, who is chasing the effects of aging by building up muscles in older adults through emphasizing the "eccentric" phase of weightlifting. For example, when you bench-press barbells, there are two phases of the exercise: the concentric phase, in which you press against gravity, and the eccentric phase, in which you lower the barbell with the help of gravity. Evans believes that this latter "easy" phase is as least as important in building muscle mass as grunting against gravity. The really good news discovered by the Tufts University team is that once the initial ten-week program was completed, working out on the weights even once a week maintained and even improved the physical ability of the ninety-something-year-old adults. Even two years after the initial program, these seniors were just as physically able to walk and climb stairs as they had been after completing the concentrated ten-week program.

For individuals not wishing to join an exercise gym, a weight bench with an attached knee exerciser and accomanying weight set can be purchased for $75 to $100 at discount stores. Obviously, the bench must be sturdy; this is much more important than having a number of costly attachments that may never be used.

Individuals attempting weight training should either do it under the guidance of a trained instructor or very carefully follow the instructions given with the exercise equipment. It is possible to do both muscle and structural damage by attempting to move too quickly from a sedentary lifestyle to an Arnold Schwarzenegger–type workout.

3. *Isokinetic exercise* (work those pecs!). Isokinetic exercises are very much like isotonic, except that exertion is required both going from the starting position and then returning to it. Generally speaking, this form of exercise requires special equipment, such as a Nau-

tilus machine, in which the individual can adjust the tension according to his or her level of training. This kind of exercise is not only expensive, but it's also inconvenient, in that it requires the individual to belong to a health club in order to use its equipment. But for those individuals who like the social atmosphere of a gym, this might be something they'd enjoy. Unfortunately, taken by itself, it does not provide a complete exercise program.

4. *Anaerobic exercise* (no sweat). As the name implies, anaerobic exercise does not require an overall increase in the consumption of oxygen. Many everyday activities fall into this category. Exercises such as certain calisthenics, playing Frisbee in the backyard, bouncing up stairs two at a time, running to the copy machine, hailing a cab in New York City, playing softball, and other activities requiring short but rather intensive bursts of energy are considered anaerobic. Clearly, this is not a complete exercise program, in that it does nothing to increase overall cardiovascular and respiratory fitness. The benefit of such exercises is that they are often fun, which is a major reason to engage in them.

5. *Aerobic exercise* (gasp). As the name implies, aerobic exercise requires an increase in the amount of oxygen used by the body. For aerobic exercise to be effective, it must be performed over a prolonged length of time, preferably twenty to thirty minutes at submaximal effort. The most common forms of this exercise are running, jogging, and formal aerobic workouts. Other forms of aerobic exercise can, however, be equally beneficial. Rapid walking and bicycling are other examples of aerobic exercise that can be performed by nearly everyone. For walking, all that's needed is a good pair of comfortable walking shoes. For people living in congested areas such as cities, walking, as well as running, during rush hour can be quite harmful, due to the pollution from rush-hour traffic. It is recommended that any exercise in which oxygen consumption is significantly increased be performed away from polluted areas.

The five exercises we have discussed all have positive benefits for physical fitness. Combinations of two or three of them, with aerobics being one of these, would be the ideal. The key to any exercise program is to enjoy it.

Besides the obvious benefit of fitness, another plus of exercising, especially in uncrowded areas, is the exhilaration we get by being in the beauty of our natural surroundings. Listen to Jeanette, as she describes her walks around the beach:

> One of the greatest pleasures in my life is walking briskly along the beach, espcially during the early morning hours as the sun begins its ascent. The beauty of my surroundings and the feel of the warm breeze on my body fill me with a calmness that I have not experienced anywhere else. The steady pounding and crashing of the waves block out all my cares and worries and for a while I am lost in my own thoughts. As I walk along the shoreline, the sand shifts underfoot and tickles my feet; I feel like a little girl again. Gone are the worries and stresses of everyday life; my body, mind, and spirit are rejuvenated in the presence of God and nature.

Clearly, walking is much more than a physical exercise for many. It is a cleansing of the mind and soul and allows us to rejoice in the beauty of life. The words of the following Navajo prayer express this sentiment in a most eloquent manner:

> Happily may I walk,
> No longer sore may I walk,
> Impervious to pain may I walk,
> With lightness of body may I walk.

The words seem to echo the modern belief that exercise produces endorphins, which are both euphoric and analgesic. We will return to this concept later, as we further examine the physiological relationship between exercise and mood.

Exercises such as bicycling and cross-country skiing are also aerobic exercises that allow us to delight in the beauty of planet Earth. Lois, a cyclist, describes her pleasure in cycling in the out-of-doors:

> Any aerobic exercise releases endorphins in your brain. That works in the short term, but cycling also takes you out into nature and helps your soul. It changes my whole perspective on life. I've never been on a ride I'm sorry I took.

But let's face it, there are many people whose purpose in undertaking an exercise program is primarily to reduce their weight rather than to enhance their overall health or to achieve euphoria through communing with nature. Happily, unless the desire to lose weight is pathological, these benefits are closely related. A loss of excess body fat will nearly always lead to better health and an improved sense of well-being. Obviously, the body's repository of excess fat (rather than muscle) is the appropriate target of weight-loss programs. To discover how different kinds of exercise can lead to the maximum loss of body fat, we need to learn some basic truths about the physiology of exercise.

Exercise requires energy in order to propel the muscles of the body. This comes from a molecule known as adenosinetriphosphate (ATP), which releases energy as it breaks down during exercise. After breaking down, ATP must then be regenerated in order for the muscles to continue working. The fuel that the body uses to regenerate ATP is either fats or carbohydrates. This fuel is burned in the body by using oxygen, just as a stove uses oxygen to burn coal or wood. Fats and carbohydrates are completely consumed under aerobic (oxygen-rich) conditions to produce carbon dioxide and water. Fat, however, has more than twice the fuel capacity (nine calories per gram) of carbohydrates (4 calories per gram). Although fat has more calories, it burns more slowly than carbohydrates during exercise, just as coal burns more slowly than wood, but releases more total energy. While you are simply puttering around the house or gardening, you do not have a high energy demand. During these activities, fat is the primary source of energy consumed to regenerate ATP. But if you start jogging or running, you suddenly need more energy and more oxygen to supply your muscles with ATP. Because you need more energy immediately, the body quickly shifts from burning fat to burning carbohydrates, such as glucose or glycogen (a starchlike substance stored in the liver). Carbohydrates produce ATP faster but less efficiently than fat in terms of the calories contained per gram.

Normally, the body has two to four hours of carbohydrate stored in glycogen for vigorous exercise. After this glycogen is gone, or even before it is completely gone, the exerciser will begin to falter and be unable to continue the pace. Marathoners and long-distance cyclists call this experience of glycogen deficiency "hitting the wall." The individual has pushed him- or herself until all of the stored glycogen in the muscles and the liver is nearly exhausted. At this time, the primary fuel available to continue is fat. As indicated, fat burns very slowly, and an individual is unable to continue vigorous running or cycling by burning fat alone.

Individuals who hit the wall will stagger about and sometimes collapse. Running to this level of carbohydrate depletion is extremely dangerous, since the brain itself needs glucose (a carbohydrate) in order to function. To avert depletion of glycogen during the race, marathoners stuff themselves with pasta and other forms of carbohydtates for several days before running a marathon. The goal is to build up a supply of glycogen in the muscles and in the liver in order to minimize the chances of hitting the wall.

Sandy had not run a marathon for some time when she first began to train for an upcoming race. The night before the marathon, she and a friend were at a dinner party where considerable amounts of protein, in the form of fish, and carbohydrates, in the form of rice, were served. Her friend, thinking of the upcoming marathon, urged Sandy to eat more rice and less fish. Yet, as the fish was exceedingly good, Sandy proceeded to ignore the rice, which is rich in carbohydrates, and ate primarily fish. Her friend described the race:

> The next day, during the race, I went back to a point about four or five miles from the finish line to cheer Sandy on as she ran past. I saw her about 300 yeards away and I knew immediately that something was wrong. She was not running with her usual confident and strong stride. I quickly hurried back to the finish and arrived just as she crossed the line and collapsed. Fortunately, as she was in superb physical condition, she was soon revived.

Although not many of us will be running marathons, hopefully all of us will be involved in some program of healthful exercise. Can we use present knowledge of physiology to achieve our optimum physical state? Let's return to the bout of vigorous running you undertook after puttering around in the garden. As you begin to run, fat consumption drops dramatically, because it is slow to furnish energy. Carbohydrate consumption increases dramatically, as it burns faster than fats and can immediately furnish the energy needed for the larger demand from the muscles. At this point in the aerobic process, the body, by necessity, is consuming carbohydrates much more rapidly than fat. In fact, the consumption of carbohydrates will increase to about 85 percent of total energy consumed almost immediately after one begins to run, and use of fat will fall dramatically. After a short period of time (twenty to thirty minutes), however, if the initial pace if not too fast (slow jogging or fast walking), the consumption of fat now begins to rise slowly. As you continue exercising, the body will attempt to conserve carbohydrates (glycogen) and begin to burn fat more efficiently. Provided the intensity of the exercise is below maximal, consumption of fat exceeds carbohydrate consumption after about thirty to forty minutes. At the end of an hour, fat consumption will be much more prevalent than carbohydrate consumption. This is the typical pattern of energy supplied during an aerobics class or a five- to ten-mile jog. Another added benefit, and a bona fide motivator for strenuous exercise, is that you will continue burning both fat and carbohydrates even after you have stopped exercising. The longer you exercise, the longer you will continue to burn calories after you have quit the exercise.

It should be very clear that longer periods of submaximal aerobic exercise are more productive than shorter periods of more intense anaerobic exercise. As illustrated by the running example, during the more intense maximal exercise, the body's demand for energy is so great that it cannot be furnished by fat and the body will burn primarily carbohydrates. With exercise less intense than running, such as rapidly walking, the body soon converts from carbohydrate consumption to fat consumption. In other words, if your exercise intensity is below maximum, the efficiency of oxygen use is high, and this permits the body to utilize fat for fuel as opposed to using carbohydrates. Conversely, if your workout is extremely intense, as you approach your maximum oxygen uptake, your consumtpion of fats will decrease and the consumption of glycogen will increase. Therefore, three workouts of an hour or so at lower intensity will burn more fat than six workouts of thirty minutes or so at a higher intensity. In addition, high-intensity exercises are more likely to result in muscular or skeletal injury.

The bottom line is that not everyone needs to be a Frank Shorter in order to be physically fit. The myth that one must "go for the burn" and experience "no pain, no gain" is just not true and keeps what may otherwise be motivated people on the couch.

Now that we know how the body needs carbohydrates as well as fats to fuel our aerobic body, how can we use this information to devise a suitable exercise program?

Exercise for Body Trimming

O, that this too too solid flesh would melt, thaw and resolve itself into a dew!

—*William Shakespeare, Hamlet*

It is certainly true that not everyone is, or should be, satisfied with his or her present body weight. For these individuals, exercise offers a mechanism but not a guarantee of success; tenacity and dedication do. It is sad but true that the body gives up its pound (or even ounce) of fat very grudgingly. The body's conservation of fat is an evolutionary survival mechanism, resulting from its experience with periods of food deprivation. For early humans, it was equally important for survival that the stored body fat not be depleted too rapidly, even when normal activity was maintained. The fact that you are here today is due in great measure to the large amount of energy (9 calories per gram) stored in fat. The bad news is that to reduce your weight by 1 gram (454 grams are equal to 1 pound), you need to burn at least this amount (1 gram) of fat. Table 6.1 lists the amount of calories expended during various exercises.

This table gives the discouraging news. Exercise, even hard exercise, does not burn many calories. If your sole purpose is to lose body fat, the facts are even worse than the table indicates.

As we have seen, the aerobically active body needs to burn carbohydrates, as well as fat. Remember that, for about thirty minutes into your exercise workout, you are burning more calories in the form of carbohydrates than fat. It is only after this time that fat calories are being consumed in greater amounts. Even more discouraging is the fact that even if you are burning equal calories from fat and carbohydrates, you must expend more than twice as many calories to consume 1 pound of fat as those needed to consume 1 pound of carbohydrates.

Assuming that your exercise program consumes 50 percent of total calories as fat and 50 percent as carbohydrates (which furnish less than one-half the calories of fat), walking for one hour at 3¾ miles per hour would burn off 150 calories of fat at 9 calories per gram or less than 0.04 pounds (there are 68 calories in a slice of bread). Put in practical terms, you would need to walk twenty-five

TABLE 6.1

*Approximate Energy Expenditure by a 150-Pound Person
in Various Activities*

Activity	Calories Expended per Hour
Lying down or sleeping	80
Sitting	100
Driving an automobile	120
Standing	140
Domestic work	180
Walking, 2½ mph	210
Bicycling, 5½ mph	210
Gardening	220
Golf, lawn mowing with power mower	250
Bowling	270
Walking, 3¾ mph	300
Swimming, ¼ mph	300
Square dancing, volleyball, roller skating	350
Wood chopping or sawing	400
Tennis	420
Skiing, 10 mph	600
Squash, handball	600
Bicycling, 13 mph	660
Running, 10 mph	900

Source: Based on material prepared by Robert E. Johnson, M.D., Ph.D., and colleagues, University of Illinois, House and Garden Bulletin No. 232, Departments of Agriculture and Health and Human Services.

times at this speed to burn off 1 pound of fat. Pretty depressing, isn't it?

But don't despair yet! As Yogi Berra said, "It ain't over till it's over," and it isn't over yet. We have seen that the body continues to consume calories, even after we stop exercising. Even more important is that regular conditioning of our body creates additional muscle tissue that must be supplied with energy on a more or less continuing basis. This is an additional value of a lifelong program of exercise for those of us who have picked our parents poorly and have a genetic predisposition to be overweight. Exercise also has been shown to lower the set-point, the point below which it is nearly impossible to lose weight, regardless of how much we diet. Detail will be included on this subject later, as we discuss the struggle to lose weight through dieting.

Clearly, the most effective way to shape up our bodies including enhancing muscle tone and reducing fat, is to combine a sensible exercise program with an equally sensible diet. It is critical for each person to choose an exercise program that fits into his or her life-style and is consistent with his or her personal preferences. If the exercise is not enjoyable, it is not likely to be continued for a significant amount of time. Obviously, one's life is not enhanced if attempts to remain healthy consist of episodic bouts of dreaded drudgery. If you don't like running, don't do it. Do something else: play tennis, bike, walk, golf, play handball, ski, and so forth.

Integrating Exercise in Your Daily Routine

Exercise, like the rest of life, should be fun, not a painful struggle to be endured. What are we living for, if we merely endure in a grim state of joyless existence?

Joyce Brothers asks the question, "Do we have enough fun?" and proceeds to answer it in the negative. She lists eleven ways to increase our fun. Ten of these can be applied directly to exercise.

1. *Get lost in the moment.* Whether you're walking along the beach like Jeanette or cycling like Lois, you should focus on the moment and leave your troubles behind. Don't be concerned: they will still be there when you return.
2. *Be incomparable.* Don't compare yourself to others when you exercise. If you can't run like Sandy, so what? Hopefully, you are exercising for health and happiness, not to look like Michelle Pfieffer.
3. *Accept yourself.* You have the body you have. You can make it healthy and strong, but you can't grow taller (or shorter). Work to improve what Nature gave you, not to completely change it. Most of us are not going to look like Arnold Schwarzenegger or Cher, and to attempt to do so defeats the purpose of a sensible exercise program.
4. *If you don't enjoy it, don't do it.* If your exercise is drudgery, you probably will soon give it up, as do a large percent of people who start exercise programs.

5. *Get off the sidelines and into the game.* Stop thinking about getting started; turn off the TV and start. Do something, even if it's just a brisk walk around the block for a starter. If you have trouble getting organized for this walk, here's a simple solution: put down this book and walk out the door. Now!

6. *Variety counts.* In exercise, as in fun (or even more, in life), it is important to vary your activities, even if this means walking a different route once in a while, taking up a new sport, or climbing a different mountain.

7. *Couples: play together and stay together.* It is much more fun to exercise with a significant other or a good friend. You also encourage each other to get moving. In today's impersonal world, however, it may be difficult to find such a person who is willing to accompany you on your routine. Don't let this deter you. Just do it, even if you do it alone.

8. *Avoid falling into a rut.* If some Wednesday morning you don't feel like exercising, even though you are supposed to every Wednesday, don't. Skipping one day won't turn you into a blubber-ox. Exercise should be fun; if you overritualize it, it could become boring.

9. *Don't overschedule.* Don't plan so much exercise into an already tight schedule that you begin to resent the time spent exercising.

10. *Don't just sit there, either.* Perhaps you should reexamine your schedule and eliminate those activities which are not really important, rather than cutting back on exercise or resenting the time spent in strengthening your body. What about getting up earlier? Dan, the college administrator mentioned earlier, gets up between 4:00 and 5:00 A.M. to get in his forty-five to sixty minutes of varied exercise.

The Personal Pleasure Inventory should be useful in helping you to select an exercise program that is both enjoyable and beneficial. For example, if spending time outdoors and enjoying nature is a natural high, why not consider running, walking, cycling, cross-country skiing, or playing tennis, rather than an aerobics class or game of racquetball? Most people live within a short distance of places where at least walking, running, and cycling are available. For walking and running, be certain to have suitable shoes, not necessarily the latest and most expensive model. If at all possible, avoid running on cement; choose blacktop or dirt. As with all exercise programs, spend a few minutes warming up before beginning the exercise in earnest. Also, if you have spent a lifetime of inactivity, see your physician before beginning a serious exercise program.

Now that we have all this information, can we really spot-trim those thighs or spot-reduce that belly? *Unfortunately, not exactly.* Then why bother with all this huff-and-puff? Why not just become a dedicated couch potato? The answer is that you can reduce total body fat but not spot-reduce. Throw away the Thighmaster and start walking! The Thighmaster may firm thigh muscles, but it cannot specifically reduce the amount of fat on your thighs. Reduction of fat is a *total* body process, and unfortunately, fat is much easier to put on than to take off. Both diet and exercise will reduce body fat, but extreme dieting can be dangerous, due to loss of lean body tissue as well as fat. On the other hand, exercise increases lean body tissue (muscle) while reducing fat tissue.

The benefits obtained by improving our bodies is only the icing on the cake of a physically active lifestyle. While an attractive body may benefit us in the "amor" department, another benefit for "long life and happiness" is in the effect of exercise on *salud,* health. It is really true that exercise can enhance the health of not only those with diseases but also those who are disease-free? Just as important, can exercise not only improve health, but prevent disease? And finally, will exercise enhance longevity? The answer to all three questions is, Absolutely!

Run for Your Life: Ponce de León Revisited

It has been said that the human body is the only machine that wears out when not used. Probably no single factor is so important to your health as a sensible program of exercise. According to the *Journal of the American Medical Association,* people with active lifestyles are far less likely to die from cancer and heart disease than their physically out-of-shape contemporaries. For physically active men, the decrease in deaths from heart disease was more than eight times that of those who did not exercise. For women, the mortality rate was seven times less for the active women.

In a series of studies, Ralph Paffenbarger of the Stanford University School of Medicine tested the following factors on the risk of coronary heart disease: blood pressure, body mass, physical activity, cigarette smoking, history of hypertension, and family history of hypertension and heart attacks. Of all these factors, physical inactivity ranked ahead of all except hypertension as a predictor of coronary heart disease (CHD).

The health benefits of physical activity were found to be independent of all the other variables tested. For example, inactive men who had a history of hypertension and smoked (a deadly combination often called "suicide in the fast lane") had a rate of CHD more than twice that of physically active smokers. Research has also shown that moderate aerobic exercise may eliminate the need for drug therapy in treating mild hypertension. Here's more good news: CHD not only can be slowed, but it can be reversed, without drugs. What better gift to yourself and your loved ones than to add years of healthy living to your life. Yes, it's true: we can live longer by exercising. In a later study, Paffenbarger showed that not only can we be healthier through physical activity, but longevity, too, can be extended. Other studies have shown that even mild, routine exercises of twenty minutes or more, done at least three times a week, can add healthy years to our lives. In his search for the Fountain of Youth, Ponce de León should have taken up jogging, rather than sloshing through the Everglades of Florida.

Probably the research hardest for you to believe is that involving the inverse relationship between exercise and cancer. But it's true—physical activity has been shown to protect against cancer of all types. Studies by the Institute of Aerobic Research showed that deaths from all cancers were approximately four times greater for the male couch potatoes and more than four times greater for the female soap-opera watchers compared to those for their physically fit contemporaries.

Martha Slattery at the University of Utah found that various types of physical activity protected against colon cancer and that women benefited more than men in this protective effect.

Another obvious advantage of physical activity among post-menopausal women is reduced risk of osteoporosis. Bones react against loss of mass by putting weight on them through exercise such as walking, running, biking, or weight training.

C. J. Caspersen and co-workers reviewed the literature on the effect of physical activity in preventing disease in healthy adults. They concluded that exercise was a beneficial prophylactic in preventing CHD, obesity, hypertension, osteoporosis, and non-insulin-dependent diabetes. Some have taken the healing power of exercise to a fine art or, alternatively, to what might be considered an extreme, depending on your viewpoint. A recent book published by Rodale Press recommends specific exercises for particular diseases or disorders. Precise exercises to ward off aging, help lower cholesterol, prevent colds, cure constipation, enhance memory, increase sexual enjoyment, eliminate anxiety, cure headaches, relieve PMS, enhance sleep, release emotionally stabilizing neurotransmitters, and prevent blood clots are only a few of the many exercises that are recommended. While we do not discourage such exercise plans, we feel that overall physical fitness accomplished by combining two or more of the five types we have discussed is the best preventive of physical disease and emotional strain. This is especially true if aerobic exercise is part of the program.

By now, you must be saying, "Come on, now, get a grip! Exercise protects me against cancer, heart disease, and hypertension, OK, I believe it, possibly even diabetes, if we're overweight, and even osteoporosis. But colon cancer? No way!" It does seem incredible that something as simple and easy to do as exercise could have so many positive benefits for health. Yet the evidence is indisputable: exercise does lead to better body image, better health, and greater longevity.

Optimal Health and the Immune System

In order to understand how exercise can be such a powerful stimulus for optimal living, we need to know something about how our bodies have evolved to maintain a wholeness in the presence of environmental assaults that might be expected to diminish our vitality.

In the first place, we need to understand that health is not defined by the number of diseases that we do not have. In fact, many people who do not have "diseases" are in ill health. We further believe that health and not illness is the "normal" human condition. The human body has marvelous built-in mechanisms for remaining well, in spite of daily attacks by foreign organisms and toxic chemicals. We are bombarded daily with foreign substances that could prove fatal if left unchallenged. The guardian of our physical well-being is known as the immune system, which, unlike a centralized unit, such as the brain, is spread throughout the body. If a foreign body such as a virus or bacteria (known as antigens) invades our body, one component of the immune system springs into action by producing molecules known as antibodies, which combine with these foreign bodies to deactivate them. Many other foreign bodies (besides viruses and bacteria), such as chemicals, are not fatal in themselves, but, if undetected, may bring about alterations in cellular chemistry that in turn result in diseases such as cancer. Many of these toxins may slip past the immune system's first line of defense, and antigen-antibody complex. Yet we ingest millions of potentially toxic molecules daily without experiencing disease. Although the immune system initially fails to recognize many of these cancer-causing molecules, our "guardian angels" are not indifferent to the effect these chemicals may have on our bodies. Should these toxins subsequently produce cancer cells, our immune system has the ability to recognize them as cancer cells and destroy them before they gain a foothold. Clearly, to remain well, we must have a strong immune system. The tragedy of AIDS is that the HIV virus somehow slowly destroys this complex "guardian angel" system and allows "criminal" elements to attack healthy cells at will.

Although AIDs is an extreme example of what happens when the immune system itself is attacked, many other diseases (e.g., cancer and pneumonia) can result if this system is even slightly damaged. We believe that one very important determinant in such a weakening of the immune system and therefore a major cause of disease is stress, something we all experience almost daily. (See Chapter 4 for major life stressors and psychological means for stress reduction.) If we are to experience maximum pleasure through sound bodies and healthy minds, we must develop body awareness skills to complement the stress-busting attributes of optimism, personal calm, and creative lifestyle described in Chapters 4 and 5. Let's consider the effect of stress on our bodies.

The volume of research on the relationship between stress and disease increases daily. Stress has been shown to be a risk factor or exacerbator in disorders such as cardiovascular disease, hypertension, cancer, streptococcal diseases, gastrointestinal disorders, tuberculosis, and a cast of other maladies. Studies of both humans and animals have shown a positive relationship between various types of stress and diminishing function of the immune system. While much research needs to be done, it seems certain that (1) a strong immune system is needed to maintain optimal wellness, and (2) excessive stress may jeopardize health by weakening the immune system.

Most scientists believe that the immune system is the mediator between stress and disease. This is not surprising, since the immune system and the central nervous system, which is involved in stress, share many features. Although at present there is not absolute proof, we are convinced that there is a three-way linkage between stress, the immune system, and compromised health. In fact, a new branch of science known as psychoneuroimmunology has recently emerged, and has as its focus the study of the relationship between the central nervous system and the immune system. It is only a matter of time before indisputable evidence for a definite link between stress, the specific immune system, and disease will be found.

A similar problem exists with the research dealing with the effect of exercise on the immune system. Since exercise clearly promotes optimal health, we would expect exercise to show a strengthening of the immune system. In all scientific reports, this has not been the case. In most of the research, however, only certain portions of the immune system were studied. Even more significant is that most studies deal with immediate alterations in the immune system following acute bouts of exercise, such as rigorous running or cycling. Obviously, protection against disease does not occur as the result of a sudden burst of aerobic exercise; rather, it is built up over a long period, during which exercise composes a major component of a totally healthy lifestyle.

Nonetheless, it is not important to belabor the reader with the available evidence for a nondisputable linkage between exercise and the immune system. What we are really interested in is the effect of exercise on stress, that all-too-common, modern-day malady that diminishes our lives at every opportunity. Since stress has been shown unequivocally to be a significant factor in disease, we are very interested in the exercise-stress-disease linkage.

Exercise versus Stress

Since most scientific evidence points to the close linkage between stress and disease, any activity that reduces mental anxiety would certainly be of benefit in enhancing both our physical and mental well-being. Could exercise be such a factor in the reduction of stress? The scientific world answers this question with a resounding *yes*. Every study on the effect of exercise (especially those exercises which aim toward maintaining general physical fitness) on stress and general mental health has been positive. This beneficial effect on mental health, as well as general mood elevation, has been observed across a wide population, ranging from the severely depressed to those whom we would consider mentally sound.

Stress is such a general term that it includes many neuronal aberrations. One of the first to study the effect of exercise on anxiety was William Morgan and co-workers at the University of Wisconsin. In the 1970s, they showed that exercise could reduce anxiety levels in almost all subjects, even those who were not especially "stressed-out." These researchers also used volunteers who underwent acute bouts of exercise, rather than regular physically fit exercisers, as the yardstick for anxiety reduction.

Temporary reduction of anxiety following acute maximal exercise is not a good barometer of the effect of exercise on mental health. It should be obvious that it is difficult to be depressed or anxious in the middle of a vigorous aerobic workout, in which your most immediate concern is getting enough oxygen to keep you going. This type of research presents no surprise; nor is it especially useful in understanding the effect of exercise in enhancing long-term optimal living. After all, how many of us can go for a three-mile run every time we become anxious about some problem in the office or factory? On the other hand, research has shown tht acute strenuous exercise is helpful in reducing what is known as "state anxiety," which is a temporary condition brought on by a specific distressful situation, such as an office squabble or a fight with your spouse or lover. So a brief run after such an episode could be helpful, provided, of course, that your general physical condition allows you to do this.

Most of us are troubled from time to time by the aforementioned kind of transient malaise when there is a feeling that everything is going wrong, but which disappears when the situation improves. In addition, many of us tend to have a bit of "trait anxiety," which is a general and somewhat persistent personality characteristic. We would very much like to know how to innoculate ourselves against attacks of both trait and state anxiety. These attacks can rob us of the chance for maximum wellness, which we all deserve.

Carlyle Folkins of the University of California at Sacramento showed that people who exercise over a long period, and at least three times per week, have significantly lower levels of anxiety and depression than nonexercisers. Even more encouraging is the work of Bonita Long of the University of British Columbia, who took three groups of stressed "couch potatoes" (i.e., their lifestyles were sedentary—no exercise) and divided them into three groups: (1) one group took up jogging; (2) another group underwent stress innoculation (meditation) training; and (3) the control group stayed on the wait list, that is, the couch. All groups were measured for trait and state anxiety following the ten-week test period and after a twelve-week and a fifteen-month follow up. Both the jogger and the stress innoculation groups tested lower on both of these forms of anxiety than the control group, even after fifteen months. Most of us face frustrating, anxiety-producing situations every day but consider ourselves normal, certainly not clinically depressed. The research to date clearly indicates that habitual exercisers suffer less from everyday depression than nonexercisers. Further, marathoners are significantly more mentally healthy than regular joggers, who, in turn, suffer less from depression than nonexercisers. These findings hold for people of different ages and for different ethnic groups. It seems that running or engaging in any other aerobic activity at least three times per week might be a good alternative or at least an adjunct to psychoanalysis for many people, and it would be cheaper. Even very expensive jogging shoes can be obtained for around $75 (one hour of psychotherapy), less on sale. If you pay more than this, you are paying for more than comfortable foot support, but that's your option, just as is buying the latest in running outfits to impress other similarly clad and shod joggers.

So now you are convinced that exercise can help ward off anxiety and other forms of stress. You should also be convinced that by reducing stress, regular exercise provides excellent protection against such devastating diseases as cancer, hypertension, heart disease, obesity, and diabetes. But what about that miserable cold or the general "blahness" that plagues us regularly and robs us of much pleasure in life?

Optimal health is not necessarily defined by the absence of cataclysmic diseases such as those mentioned. In fact, most people who seek medical attention do not have any of these or any other disease, but are not in good health. General lack of good health in our citizens constitutes a major economic problem for this country. People in chronic ill health (with no definable disease) spend an average of seven days a month in bed. Stress has been associated with nonspecific ill health in a number of scientific studies. In one study, N. Beale and co-workers found that the stress of a threatened or actual job loss was associated with a 70 percent increase in episodes of illness, a 150 percent increase in medical consultations, and a 200 percent increase in attendance at outpatient departments. Another example, but less stressful than loss of a job, is exam time for college students. Obviously, students need to be extra sharp and in top physical condition during this period. Unfortunately, stress-related illnesses such as flu, sore throats, colds, and other infectious diseases, as well as stomach disorders, seem to increase during this time. Nearly all studies indicate that exercise can protect against these stress-related illnesses. This immunity, however, seems to be conferred only on those who maintain physical fitness as a way of life, not on those who practice the frantic frenzy of a two-month crash program.

Research by David Sinyor at Concordia University showed that even an exercise program lasting for ten weeks failed to confer any appreciable protection against stress-related alterations in heart rate. Although the alterations in heart rate were not correlated to any specific disease or illness, this research does confirm our thesis that optimal living through reduction of stress is not a quick fix but a lifelong commitment.

There seems to be no doubt that physical fitness alleviates most major stress-related symptoms, but what about that "gray drizzle of horror," depression, which robs the victim of any hope for a satisfying life and robs the U.S. economy of more than $16 billion per year in medical costs and lost productivity?

Running Away from Depression

Opposite to Exercise is Idleness or want of exercise, the bane of body and mind . . . and a sole cause of Melancholy.
—*Robert Burton, 1632*

Although the scientific study of the relationship between a healthy mind and exercise is recent, through the years it has been recognized that lack of exercise is a deterrent to happiness.

In 1978, J. H. Griest at the University of Wisconsin found that a regimen of regular jogging reduced symptoms in a group of depressed outpatients more than a regimen of psychotherapy did. Even more encouraging was the one-year follow-up, which found that most of the members of the running group had become regular runners and had remained symptom-free. Since that time, dozens of studies have been conducted on the effect of both acute (usually single aerobic events) and chronic (long-term physical fitness) exercise. In nearly all cases, exercise, even anaerobic exercise, was found to be beneficial in reducing symptoms of depression. One study showed that exercise was as effective as group psychotherapy or individual psychotherapy, and a lot less expensive.

One problem not addressed by some of these early studies is that of self-selection for exercise. Could it be that motivated people who exercise are naturally less depressed, while depressed people lack the motivation to exercise? The difference is critical if we are to recommend exercise as a prescription for our everyday lives, which are often troubled by occasional depressive episodes. Although exercise clearly helped those in Griest's early study of clinically depressed patients, will beginning a program of exercise benefit those of us who up until now have not chosen exercise as a part of our lives? Griest's more recent experiment showed this to be the case. He randomly assigned depressed patients to one of three groups: individuals involved in aerobic exercise, those taking relaxation training, or those receiving group psychotherapy. After twelve weeks, all three groups showed improvement, but after three months, only the exercise group and the relaxation group continued to improve.

As encouraging as these results may be for these patients, they do not necessarily relate to most of us, who are not clinically depressed but do have occasional episodes of mild depression that often rob us of some of life's joys. Most research indicates that exercise can help us rid ourselves of the often too frequent "blahs." I. L. McCann at the University of Kansas randomly assigned a group of mildly depressed female students at the University of Kansas to three groups: (1) an aerobic exercise group; (2) a group that practiced muscle relaxation; and (3) a no-treatment group. At the end of ten weeks, only those in the aerobic group showed dramatic decreases in depression. Nearly every study since has confirmed that exercise provides excellent protection against depression.

So it seems that exercise, especially long-term aerobic exercise, is an excellent prophylactic against stress, anxiety, and both mild and clinical depression.

Healthy Body, Healthy Mind

The natural healing force within us is the greatest force in getting well.
—*Hippocrates*

By now, you must be thinking that we're pushing exercise as a modern-day "snake oil" medicine-show remedy for nearly every physical ailment, as well as for various mental afflictions, such as stress, anxiety, and depression. Hopefully, you are convinced of the rather obvious effect of overall physical fitness on such major illnesses as diabetes, obesity, heart disease, and hypertension. We also hope you are at least considering the possibility that protection against cancer can be achieved by exercise-induced strengthening of the immune system. But stress, depression, and anxiety are mental, not physical, right? Granted, the mind can affect the body, but can the reverse be true? For example, we know that a healthy mind free from stress promotes good bodily health, but can a healthy body produce a healthy mind? Can there actually be a connection between bodily fitness and mental health? Clearly, this concept is not new. Holistic medicine, which regards the mind and body as a single entity, has been a belief of Hindu philosophy for centuries. As we have seen, most modern research clearly indicates a definite correlation between these two. But how does it work? In order to understand this connection, we need to look more closely at the mind-body connection, mentioned previously as the hypothalamus-pituitary-adrenal (HPA) axis, represented schematically in Figure 6.1.

In response to outside stimuli, including stress, higher centers in the brain, such as the hippocampus, relay messages to the hypothalamus, that portion of the brain which regulates emotion, as well as many other basic processes of life, such as eating and body temperature. The hypothalamus then relays the stress signals by sending certain chemicals (CRF) to the pituitary gland, which lies at the base of the brain. This gland then releases other molecules, including endorphins and ACTH, which in turn alert the outer layer (cortex) of the adrenal glands, which are situated on top of the kidneys. The

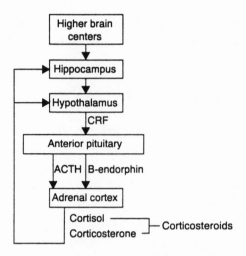

The Hypothalamus-Pituitary-Adrenal (HPA) Axis

Stressful stimuli are relayed to a portion of the hypothalamus, which
responds by releasing CRF, which then activates the pituitary. This
activation causes this gland to release ACTH and Bendorphin. The
former (ACTH) causes increased synthesis of corticosteroids, which
bring about the release of adrenaline and norepinephrine.
Negative feedback mechanisms from the adrenal cortex to the
hippocampus and the hypothalamus constitute part of the system's
homeostatic regulating mechanism.

adrenal cortex secretes other molecules, known as corticosteroids,
such as cortisol, which control a number of body functions. These
include preparing the body for an emergency by releasing adrenaline
and norepinephrine. As in all bodily, as well as mental, functions,
there are regulating mechanisms which work toward achieving homeostasis. In our HPA system, one of the regulating mechanisms is
a negative feedback loop that is activated by corticosteroids, which
in turn inhibit sending the molecular message from the hypothalamus to the pituitary gland. There are other molecular organizations
that regulate the HPA system, including the now familiar neurotransmitters dopamine, norepinephrine, and serotonin, as well as
the equally familiar endorphins. Once again, it seems that these molecules literally have the power to control our lives both physically
and mentally. It is believed that in depressed people, the homeostasis
of the HPA axis is upset. It is further believed that stress can also
upset the HPA system and that continued, unrelenting stress can

lead to depression. It is also quite possible that due to the genetic basis of depression, genetically generated disregulation of the HPA system may cause depression. One study indicates that about half of depressed patients have abnormal corticosteroid levels, which are believed to have the potential to damage neurons of the hippocampus. Damage to the hippocampus could account for the poor short-term memory of many stressed and/or depressed patients. Since stress can upset HPA homeostasis and possibly lead to depression, it would seem logical that exercise, which we have shown to relieve stress, would at least alleviate depression by reestablishing homeostasis in the HPA system.

Runner's High: Fact or Fiction?

How does exercise, which has such a positive effect on mental attitude, restore homeostasis to a disregulated HPA system? There are many theories, many not completely proved or accepted by the scientific community. Since depression is a disease of the mind, it seems logical that we should look to that part of the HPA axis which lies within the brain, that is, the hypothalamus and the pituitary. These regions of the brain, like most others, use the langauge of chemistry in communication. As we have seen, the words of this language are neurotransmitters, which we now see are involved in regulation of the HPA axis. E. J. Sachar at Columbia University has proposed that the depletion of norepinephrine (NE) in the hypothalamus may bring about disruption of the HPA system and lead to depression. Other studies with humans and animals support this hypothesis. If, then, exercise is to have any effect on mood, including depression, we whould look to an increase in the level of NE as a result of exercise.

In fact, this has been shown to be true. Many studies demonstrate an increase in the levels of NE in the brains of chronically exercising mice. Other studies have implicated that exercise promotes entry of the amino acid tryptophan into the brain, where (as we have seen in Chapter 3) it forms the miracle neurotransmitter serotonin. The importance of enhanced NE and serotonin should be obvious when we recall from Chapter 3 that low levels of NE and serotonin have been implicated in depression. Equally fascinating is the fact that serotonin seems to be the neurotransmitter that activates the Reward Cascade. Therefore, release of serotonin would also be expected to enhance overall feelings of well-being and self-esteem. Happily, we don't need to be depressed to experience the positive mental benefits of exercise. Also, if exercise does increase levels of NE, we would expect to experience a mild case of mania while running. But mania is not the only feeling experienced by vigorous prolonged exercise such as running. There is a sense of serenity and euphoria that pervades our entire being. It is as if somehow our body is releasing those "keys to paradise," endorphins, which are the crucial molecules needed as final regulators of our Reward Cascade, our own antidepressant mechanism.

Most of the early work on the relationship between exercise and endorphins was done by studying the increase in blood levels of endorphins following acute exercise. Every study to date has shown that prolonged vigorous exercise produces peripheral increases in the level of endorphins. While this peripheral increase in endorphins would account for decreased pain perception following exercise, it would not be likely to account for the decrease in depression, since endorphins do not pass easily from the blood to the brain. Since it is considered "bad form" to surgically examine the brains of athletes following exercise, research has turned to animals. Michael Blake at Marquette University has shown that prolonged submaximal—and not brief, strenuous—exercise increases the level of endorphins in the brains of rats. Other studies have basically shown the same results. Let's now return to the Navajo prayer and analyze it in terms of neurotransmitter release during sustained walking.

Happily may I walk (*Mania: release of NE*)
No longer sore may I walk
Impervious to pain may I walk (*Analgesia: release of endorphins*)
With lightness of body may I walk (*Euphoria: release of endorphins*)

The interesting feature of research findings on exercise and mood is that prolonged, submaximal exercise produces endorphins, the euphoric and analgesic chemical, whereas short bouts of acute exercise produce NE, the manic neurochemical. One of us (Sunderwirth), who ran races for many years, has always claimed that running has two phases: the NE phase, followed by the endorphin phase. The first phase produces a manic state, presumably due to the release of NE in the locus coeruleus. Only after prolonged exertion does the effect of endorphins become noticeable. Listen to his description of a typical 10K race:

> As I began to run, I felt great confidence and thought to myself, "Why am I running this wimpy 10K race? With my level of fitness, I should be in the marathon. I can run forever at this pace." After about three miles, however, the mania subsided and I was wondering about my sanity at age sixty in competing with twenty- and thirty-year-olds, even in the 10K race.

Others have experienced both the exhilaration of the NE phase and the euphoria of the endorphin phase in the same run. Read the words of a runner, described in a student paper appropriately entitled "The Second, Second Wind!"

> Thirty minutes out, and something lifts. Legs and arms become light and rhythmic. My snake brain is making the best of it. the fatigue goes away, and feelings of power begin. I think I'll run twenty-five miles today. I'll double the size of the research grant request. I'll have that talk with the dean. . . .
>
> Then, sometime into the second hour comes the spooky time. Colors are bright and beautiful, water sparkles, clouds breathe, and my body, swimming, detaches from the earth. A loving contentment invades the basement of my mind, and thoughts bubble up without trails. I find the place I need to live if I'm going to live.

Now read the description of Robert, a student at a Midwestern university, as he describes the end of his daily aerobic run at 3:00–4:00 A.M.:

> All of a sudden, my throat opens up, [and] the air flows back into my lungs. All the tension in my body is released, and at that moment, a rush of power surges through my body. I can feel the tautness of every muscle in my being. I hear and feel my breath billowing out through my mouth, and I feel a moment of exhilaration. It's as if I'm looking through the eyes of a new and baptized person. And at that moment, I feel like I could run forever.

These vignettes are but minute examples of the powerful impact exercise has on our mental health and attitude. Hopefully, the preceding brief discussion of psychoneurobiology will give you some insight into how exercise exerts its beneficial effects on your disposition.

Regardless of the neurochemical mechanism involved, the undisputable evidence is that exercise does have a positive effect on mood. As long ago as 1984, the National Institute of Mental Health conducted a state-of-the-art workshop on exercise and mental health. The participants formulated the following consensus:

1. Physical fitness is positively associated with mental health and well-being.
2. Exercise is associated with the reduction of stress emotions such as state anxiety.
3. Anxiety and depression are common symptoms of failure to cope with mental stress, and exercise has been associated with a decreased level of mild to moderate depression and anxiety.
4. Long-term exercise is usually associated with reductions in traits such as neuroticism and anxiety.
5. Severe depression usually requires professional treatment, which may include medication, electroconvulsive therapy, and/or psychotherapy, with exercise as an adjunct.
6. Appropriate exercise results in reductions in various stress indices such as neuromuscular tension, resting heart rate, and some stress hormones.
7. Current clinical opinion holds that exercise has beneficial emotional effects across all ages and in both sexes.
8. Physically healthy people who require psychotropic medication may safely exercise when exercise and medications are titrated under close medical supervision.

Clearly, if you want to improve your attitude, your health, and your life, get off the couch and get going.

Make Life a Moving Experience

Actually, you don't have to be an exercise fanatic to benefit from the effects of literally getting off the couch. Edward Cooper, president of the American Heart Association, suggests a few simple ways we can increase our everyday physical movement. These simple, everyday activities may not burn many calories but do provide valuable tips for how to increase activity to make your life longer, healthier, and happier.

- Use the stairs (up and down) instead of the elevator. Start with one flight and gradually build up to more.
- Park a few blocks from the office or store and walk the rest of the way. Of if you ride on public transportation, get off a few stops early.
- Take an exercise break—get up from your desk, stretch, walk around and give your muscles and mind a chance to relax.
- Instead of snacking, take a brisk stroll around the neighborhood.
- When traveling, choose a hotel with a good exercise facility. Then use it.
- Walk wherever possible: up stairs, shopping, to a restaurant or meeting.
- Stand or walk while you talk on the phone. A cordless phone helps.
- Substitute bowling or miniature golf for a movie.
- Some physical activity can save you money: Mow the lawn and/or do your own housework.
- The next time you walk the dog, try walking a little faster and a little longer. If you don't have a pet, adopt one.
- Try "aerobic shopping." Wear walking shoes and sneak in an extra lap or two around the mall. Stretch to reach items in high places and squat or bend to look at items at floor level. If you try this in the supermarket, it will also get you out of the eye-level "impulse buying" zone.
- Throw away your video remote control. Instead of asking someone to bring you a drink, get up off the couch and get it yourself.

But good health as a major pathway to happiness is a two-sided coin. We have seen one side, exercise. Now let's flip the coin to the other side, our eating habits, and examine how they can enhance our body image, improve our physical and mental health, and provide us with one of life's greatest pleasures.

Eating as a Healthy Habit

Call it the Jetson diet: a futuristic feast of prefab pellets containing all the nourishment any 21st century citizen would want. It makes for a nice cartoon fantasy, but could people really eat this way? Not a chance. Real food is here to stay. . . .

The wisest strategy right now may be to redouble those efforts to eat more broccoli and carrots, spinach and squash.

—Anastasia Toufexis, The New Scoop on Vitamins

Many of us recall the Popeye cartoons of the 1940's at the Saturday afternoon matinee. Popeye would invariably become trapped in what appeared to be an impossible situation, such as being bound head to foot in chains and about to be pushed off a ship's plank. Then from nowhere, a can of spinach would appear. Popeye would manage to grab it with a free hand and squeeze it until it opened. As soon he had gulped down the contents, a miraculous transformation would occur: his biceps would expand until they were nearly the size of his head, and, with a mighty effort, he would break the chains and demolish his tormentors. Although no one actually believed that eating spinach could make a person as strong as Popeye, many a youngster grew up with the admonition, "Eat your spinach so you'll grow up to be strong!"

Folklore is rampant with beliefs concerning the beneficial physical and mental effects of different foods, including the belief that specific foods can cure specific ailments. For example, there are sassafras teas to "thin the blood," vegetables with roughage to cure constipation, fish to make you smart, oysters to enhance virility, chocolate to drive away those "lonesome lovesick blues," and chicken soup to cure the flu. Until recently, the medical profession paid little attention to these claims, and in most cases looked on them as something slightly worse than voodoo. In addition, too many doctors, when treating both acute and chronic ailments, traditionally ignored good nutrition as a prerequisite to good health. Certainly they would never consider specific foods a preventive measure to ward off certain diseases. In fact, nutrition as we know it today was often not considered a major component of the physician's medical training. Although this situation has changed dramatically in the past few years, we have not reached the point where the physician writes a prescription for broccoli, carrots, and cauliflower to treat colon cancer or bananas to treat high blood pressure. Yet with our present knowledge of the effect of diet on health, perhaps this is what physicians should be doing. Poor diets have been implicated in up to 50 percent of cancers, in many heart attacks, and in a host of other diseases. In fact, substandard eating and drinking habits have been implicated in six of the ten leading causes of death in the United States—heart disease, cancer, stroke, diabetes, atherosclerosis, and chronic liver disease, including cirrhosis. Maybe it's time we reexamined our Twinkie, burger, and potato chips diet.

Most young people can get away temporarily with an atrocious diet, but this changes as we age. If we are to make our Golden Years truly golden, we need to take steps long before reaching them to ensure that they're spent in robust physical and mental health. Long life without the happiness that good health can bring is not necessarily something to be desired. But most of us are able to have a healthy, pleasurable, and physically fit life well into our nineties if we are prudent in our lifestyle. Proper nutrition constitutes a major portion of this lifestyle and adds years of healthy and happy living to our lives.

It should come as no surprise that certain natural foods have medicinal value in maintaining health through prevention of specific diseases. Many of our modern medicines used to treat a wide range of physical and mental illnesses have come from plants not much different from those which compromise our daily diet. For example, for hundreds of years, the people of India used an extract of the snakeroot plant to treat mental illness. Modern chemists isolated the active ingredient, reserpine, which Nathan Kline successfully used in the 1950s to treat depressed patients. This began the present trend of treating mental disorders using chemicals. Anyone who believes that "natural" substances have no effect on the chemistry of the body or the brain would do well to look at those natural plants which produce mind-altering drugs, such as marijuana, cocaine, morphine, mescaline, lysergamide, tobacco, and psilocybin. One researcher has even commented that, for a single plant, the difference between a medicine, a poison, a hallucinogen, and a food may be a matter of quantity. While this may be an overstatement, it is clear that plants, which comprise our major food source, have a profound effect on our mental and physical health.

Although there is not complete agreement on which specific foods prevent or cure certain diseases, there is fortunately, very little disagreement on what constitutes a healthy diet.

The Saturated Fat–Cholesterol Link

Anyone who has not been in a cave for the past forty years is aware that too often, hamburgers constitute the main source of protein for America's young people. While it is true that red meat constitutes an excellent source of protein, it is also true that most red meat is loaded with saturated fats and cholesterol, that dynamic duo of heart disease. In recognition of this, the beef industry is making every effort to produce and market their product with less fat. Prized marbled steaks have gone the way of the Studebaker automobile. Even so, most nutritionists recommend no more than three 3-ounce servings (about the size of a deck of playing cards) of red meat a week. The problem is not so much the red meat per se, but the fat that comes with it. Fat can be a genuine obstacle in our quest for optimal health. It has been implicated in, among other diseases, cancer, weight gain (recall those 9 calories per gram), and coronary heart disease.

There are two types of fat, saturated and unsaturated, and they are not equally harmful. Saturated fats are found in animal fats, tropical oils such as coconut and palm oil, and products that contain chemically altered vegetable oils. Unsaturated fats are found in unaltered vegetable oils such as corn, cottonseed, olive, and peanut oils. While a healthy diet would consist of one that is low in both types of fat, *saturated* fats are especially to be avoided. The U.S. government's dietary guidelines recommend that no more than 30 percent of our total dietary calories come from fat. Many nutritionists believe that a limit of 20 to 25 percent of total calories, with saturated fats constituting no more than 7 percent, is desirable.

Why is saturated fat so deadly, and what is the chemical difference between it and unsaturated fat? Let's spend some time understanding this difference, as it is critical to understanding how to choose a healthy diet. Such knowledge is especially crucial in view of the many false and misleading claims on packaged and processed foods that can be confusing to any but the well informed.

The label "No Cholesterol" springs out at us from every corner of the supermarket. We see this pronouncement on products such as bread, oat bran, margarine, synthetic coffee creamer, vegetable-based cooking shortening, and peanut butter. Of *course* these products have no cholesterol, since for the most part, plants do not contain cholesterol; it is an animal product. Someday this label will probably appear on Diet Coke. The reason for this scam should be obvious. Most people over the age of ten are familiar with the link between high cholesterol and heart disease. Therefore, practically everyone who is not a chemist is an easy victim to the shameful deception perpetrated on the American people with the "No Cholesterol" label. Obviously, a healthy diet should be low in cholesterol, but dietary intake of cholesterol may not be as serious a health hazard as saturated fat. What the manufacturers don't tell you unless you can read and understand the list of ingredients is the amount of saturated fat in the product. And how does this relate to buildup of cholesterol in the body?

It has been known for more than twenty-five years that saturated fats raise the blood cholesterol level, especially that of the "bad" cholesterol (LDL). Therefore, the amount of saturated fat in a product may have a greater effect on blood cholesterol levels and heart disease than the actual amount of cholesterol in the product.

The saturated fat in processed food is often made by chemically treating unsaturated vegetable oil (the good fat) with hydrogen. It is then marketed as partially hydrogenated vegetable oil, but in reality, once hydrogenated, it is basically indistinguishable from the saturated fat that comes from animals. This leads to another, equally misleading label on some margarines and other cooking products: "Made from 100 Percent Corn Oil." But before you buy this product, expecting great health benefits, read the list of ingredients. Often the first is the now all-too-familiar "partially hydrogenated corn oil," a chemist's way of saying saturated fat. It is not certain that some margarines are healthier than butter, even if butter does have cholesterol. If you do buy margarine, buy the tub type, not the hard stick kind. The harder the margarine, the greater the percentage of saturated fat. Read the label and choose a margarine in which the *first* ingredient listed is vegetable oil. Also, look for the ratio of unsaturated fat to saturated fat. Choose the product that has more unsaturated than saturated fat. Research has shown that saturated fats have a significant impact on heart disease, possibly an even greater effect than dietary cholesterol.

In the early 1990s, as the Food and Drug Administration cracked down on labels such as "Lite," "Low Calorie," and "Low Fat," suddenly the word healthy began to appear on many name brands of foods. For example, what had once been artificially flavored and oversweetened ice cream was now "Healthy Ice Cream." Unfortunately, too many food processors rely on the uninformed American public to enable them to pawn off average or below-average food products as "healthy." The only way to know how much fat, sugar, salt, and calories you're eating (as well as to ensure that what you're eating is actually edible) is to learn to read and understand the names of the ingredients listed on the label. A general rule is that if you can't pronounce it, don't eat it.

Now let's turn our attention to what we should eat if we wish to enhance our mental and physical health.

Eating for Maximum Health

One of the earliest and most persistent advocates of proper nutrition in achieving and maintaining optimal health has been *Prevention* magazine, published by Rodale Press, named after the original founder. For many years the magazine was like a "voice in the wilderness," crying out against the sins of a Twinkie and Zinger diet while extolling the virtues of a high-quality diet as a prerequisite to a healthy body and sound mind. In 1991, Rodale Press published *The Healing Foods Cookbook*, in which particular foods are recommended for their preventive and their healing powers with regard to specific diseases. Diseases for which definite foods are recommended include anemia, cancer, diabetes, high blood pressure, stroke, urinary tract infections, and many others. While some may scoff at the idea of a "nutritional pharmacy," the foods advocated in *The Healing Foods Cookbook* are those with which no nutritionist could disagree.

The purpose of this chapter is not to outline a specific dietary plan but to stress the importance of healthy eating as a part of total body pampering, consisting of exercise, good nutrition, sensual pleasures, and relaxation. There are many reputable books and pamphlets giving specific instructions for following a healthy diet. For example, the October 1992 issue of *Consumer Reports* contains an excellent guide to what foods to chose for health and for guarding against the ravages of aging. A brief summary of these guidelines is given below.

1. Obtain most of your calories from complex carbohydrates, especially whole-grain cereals.
2. Eat at least seven servings of fruit and vegetables a day. (Seven!)
3. Eat more fish and poultry and less red meat.
4. Limit fats to less than 25 percent of total calories and saturated fats to less than 7 percent of daily calories.
5. Go easy on the booze—a drink or two a day at most.
6. Drink and eat low-fat or nonfat dairy products.

We have already discussed the benefits of a low-fat diet , but what about all those vegetables and whole-grain cereals? What is their value? They constitute our main source of fiber (Grandmother's "roughage"), which is an important aid in removal of waste products from the colon. Much research has shown that high-fiber diets provide protection against colon cancer as well as heart disease.

Seven servings a day of fruits and vegetables! Are they really necessary? Yes, they are, but remember, a serving is a half-cup, or a banana or an apple. Vegetables and fruits are rich in many vitamins, including C, E, and β-carotene (a precursor of vitamin A), all of which belong to a class of "good" molecules known as antioxidants, which scavenge the body looking for bad molecules called free radicals (molecules containing an unpaired electron). These free radicals are chemically reactive and assault and kill healthy cells. This cell destruction can result in cancer, cardiovascular disease, osteoporosis, and disorders of the immune system. Free radicals are also believed to be responsible for speeding up the process of aging. In addition to actually destroying cells, free radicals also wreak havoc with our cellular DNA, alter biochemical compounds, and damage cell membranes. They are superbad news and major deterrents to optimal health. But don't despair; they can be controlled. A diet rich in fruits and vegetables will furnish us with the big three guardians of our health—that is, vitamin's C, E, and β-carotene—all of which inhibit the damaging effects of free radicals.

If we're going to have to eat all these fruits and vegetables and cut down on meat, why not just become vegetarians? Doing so is probably not a good idea for most people. Although many swear by a vegetarian diet, the jury is still out on this one. Obviously, many people throughout the world, especially some Hindus in India, are strict vegetarians by choice and seem to do very well. Most evidence, however, would not lead us to believe that strict vegetarianism is the best, and certainly not the only, pathway to health.

But what is certain is that Americans eat too much meat and not enough vegetables. This low-meat diet was not always the prevailing view. One of us (Sunderwirth) played college football in the late 1940s and early 1950s. Before each game, the team would be required to eat at the team training table, where the fare consisted of a huge meal whose main entree was an enormous steak, with side dishes of mashed potatoes and gravy. No wonder the team was lucky to win even one game a season. Happily, this concept of a nutritious meal is changing.

Do We Need Vitamin Supplements?

If we eat so many fruits and vegetables, do we need to take vitamin supplements? Probably not, but who actually eats that many servings of whole grain's, fruits, and vegetables every day? Probably not many people. Let's face it—not everyone, including former president George Bush, likes broccoli. We probably don't eat enough vegetables and fruits to give us the assurance of a healthy diet. Also, many people who travel and eat out are especially at risk with regard to vitamin deficiency. Most menus at restaurants feature a meat dish as the main course, with a minuscule portion of vegetables thrown in, mostly for color. Therefore, many of us may need to take supplements, especially those which destroy free radicals: vitamins C, E, and β-carotene.

For years, physicians have parroted the worn statement "We get all the vitamins we need in our diet." Obviously, these doctors never stood in line at a fast-food emporium and watched the hamburgers, fries, and Diet Cokes pour over the counter.

Doug, a graduate student in chemistry at a Western university in the 1960s, asked his physician if he thought he needed vitamin C, since he had a rather poor diet, typical for many college students. His doctor replied rather curtly, "I'm the doctor; *I'll* tell you when you need vitamins." Two months later, Doug came back to see the doctor. His gums were tender and bleeding. The doctor took one look at him and snapped, "Now, you need vitamin C." Fortunately, modern medicine is becoming more and more aware of the need for vitamin supplements in the average American diet. So why not take vitamin supplements to be sure? They are an inexpensive insurance policy, but as in all facets of life, moderation, not excess, is prudent (e.g., too much vitamin A can cause liver damage). A word of caution: don't be fooled by the nonsense of the debate regarding "natural" versus "synthetic" vitamins. Vitamins are pure molecules, and it doesn't matter if the vitamin is synthetically manufactured by a chemical company or is extracted from rose hips. Vitamin C is vitamin C—period.

Earlier, we discussed the effect of exercise on people's mental states. Are we now saying that the foods people eat can also affect their mental state? Modern science would join Grandmother in answering this question in the affirmative.

Food for Thought

Fish can make you smart; milk and cookies put you to sleep; Twinkies turn you into a murderer; fat makes you dull; protein makes you alert; coffee makes you hyper. Many of these beliefs concerning the effect of foods on moods have turned out to have a scientific basis. Judith Wurtman at the Massachusetts Institute of Technology has spent years studying the effect of foods on the brain; some of these effects were discussed in Chapter 3. Along with many other researchers, she believes that the big three of neurotransmission (serotonin, dopamine, and norepinephrine), all of which are derived from foods, are to a large extent responsible for regulating our moods. Since norepinephrine and dopamine, which make us alert, are synthesized in the brain from the amino acids phenylalanine and tyrosine, a meal high in protein would energize us. Such a meal would include protein-rich fish, skinless chicken, or lean beef, as well as low-fat cottage cheese and yogurt, skim milk, peas, beans, or lentils. On the other hand, a meal loaded with carbohydrates from pastry or bread would enhance the formation of serotonin, which relaxes us and results in drowsiness.

If you need to be in top mental shape for long periods of time or for giving a presentation before colleagues, Wurtman believes that it is not only what you eat but how you eat that is important. Two hours before the presentation, eat a small, low-fat, high-protein meal. A heavy meal, such as that given to Sunderwirth's college football team, would make you groggy and mentally sluggish. Observe how after-dinner speakers just pick at their food, usually eating a small portion of the meat and vegetables and skipping the dessert. This at least keeps the speaker awake, even if everyone else has drifted into a serotonin-induced snooze.

Most college students preparing for exams eat all the wrong foods for maximizing their mental alertness. A study at Butler University in Indianapolis by Kathy Jesse showed the following eating patterns, which can be summarized by one student's comments, "We eat shit during finals week!"

1. Ramona drinks two 24-can cases of caffeine-free Diet Coke
2. Sue and her roommate stock up on Nacho Cheese Doritos
3. Steve eats popcorn and brownies and drinks a 32-ounce tumbler of coffee each night
4. Mike relies on Snickers bars to keep going all night
5. John consumes huge quantities of Bugles and root beer

According to Wurtman, all of these students are doing the opposite of what they should. Candy, sweets, and high-carbohydrate foods give one a temporary lift by elevating the level of glucose in the blood. This in turn elevates the level of serotonin in the brain and brings on drowsiness. Also, once the blood glucose level drops below normal due to the surge of insulin created by the candy bar, fatigue comes on very quickly. Wurtman would agree that only Brian, with a 3.95 grade point average, seems to have figured out how to stay alert during finals. He prepares for his exams before finals week, avoids high-carbohydrate snacks, and late-night studying, and gets enough rest and exercise—an important way to stay alert. It seems that the old adage "You are what you eat" is true for both physical and mental reasons.

Let's return to our earlier discussion of body image. We have seen how exercise affects our physical body as well as our mental body image. Now let's examine how our eating habits affect our body and our body image.

Healthy Eating and Body Image

Before we begin exploring the effect of healthy eating on our body, we need to consider altering our attitude toward our body. So long as we continue to believe that we should be model-thin, we will never be satisfied with our body. Look once again at Andrea. She has allowed her bathroom scale to dictate her emotional state. Andrea is not alone. In 1990, Americans spent more than $33 billion supporting weight-loss and other body-shaping businesses. Much of this is wasted on people who do not really need to lose weight, while many of those who are truly overweight make no effort to slim down. As everyone knows, slimming down is not all that easy. Those 9 calories per gram of fat are tough to burn off. Unfortunately, for those who are obsessed with a cover-model mentality, medical science is discovering what most of us already know: "diet" as we ordinarily think of it doesn't work. Too often, this type of dieting leads to "yo-yo" weight loss and gain. In one study, the National Center for Health Statistics reported that 90 percent of those who lost 25 pounds through dieting alone gained it back in two years. After seven years, only 2 percent of dieters had maintained their desired weight. Even more serious, this type of dieting may be harmful to one's overall health, which is just what the dieter was hoping to enhance by dieting. A recent study showed that yo-yo dieting (losing and gaining 10 to 25 pounds over and over) caused a 70 percent increase in heart disease among these dieters, relative to people whose weight stayed the same. Even "overweight" people whose weight remained constant fared better than the yo-yo dieters.

There is more bad news from recent scientific research. It is possible that we may be genetically predisposed to weigh more than we think we should. And that's not all. In addition, we may be unconsciously directed toward the type of food we eat by genetically or environmentally induced brain chemistry. Sarah Leibowitz of

Rockefeller University believes that our desire for different types of food resides in our brain and not in our stomach. For this reason, conscious attempts to alter these desires for certain foods often meet with failure. For example, we now believe that carbohydrate cravers are that way, to a large extent, because of their brain chemistry. Wurtman characterized certain people who had a serotonin imbalance in the brain as having carbohydrate craving obesity (CCO). Our desire for carbohydrates is also turned on by the neurotransmitter norepinephrine and the hormone cortisol, but is turned off by serotonin. On the other hand, a desire for protein is stimulated by levels of serotonin and endorphins in the brain. Finally—and here is yet more bad news—the desire for fat is turned on by several hormones and opiates. Unfortunately, this desire predominates during the evening, just when we are unlikely to exercise to burn it off. This craving is turned off by the neurotransmitter dopamine. The "set-point" combination of these neurotransmitter, hormone, and other effects is largely under genetic control. Our individual set-point has a great influence on our ability to shed weight and to keep it off. This explains why some people have a much more difficult time than others maintaining what they consider an ideal weight.

One type of weight problem that is all too common for most overweight men is the "beer belly." With regard to health, this is the most dangerous type of excessive weight, as it has been shown to increase the risk of heart attack. On the other hand, excess fat around the hips and thighs, more common in women, in not nearly so life-threatening.

Now to the good news. Yes, there is a great deal of good news regarding weight control. As you might have guessed, one path to weight control is exercise. A program of regular exercise has the ability to lower the set-point for many people, making it easier to keep the pounds off once they are gone. But aren't there other ways to lose unhealthy weight, in addition to regular exercise? Obviously, regulation of total calorie intake is an important as exercise. The equation for unwanted calories lost is as follows:

Calories lost = Calories lost through daily living (including exercise) – calories gained through food intake

If the calories lost through exercise exceed those gained through dietary intake, then there will be a net loss of calories, with a corresponding net loss in weight. On the other hand, if dietary calories exceed exercise calories, there will be a negative loss, which the body will interpret as a weight gain. Obviously, it is possible to trim unwanted fat, but not through the type of dieting so often undertaken by many Americans. The key is to alter the way we live on a daily, long-term basis. Although it is not an overnight process (or even a six-month process), the bottom line is that with a sensible program of exercise and healthy eating, most of us can enhance both our overall health and our body image. It is truly good news that the word *diet* as we commonly know it is losing acceptance in our society and is being replaced by an emphasis on overall changes in our lifestyle, including exercise and proper nutrition. The focus of the 1990s and beyond is more on being healthy than on being superthin.

"Ideal weight" charts now give much more flexibility and a wider range of "ideal" weight than previously was the case. Even so, there is great variability in bone density and muscle mass, which can cause distortion of body image if too much reliance is placed on these charts. But if you are far outside this range, either way, you need to seriously look at your exercise program and eating habits.

Believe it or not, one of our recommendations for enhancing body image and losing weight is to eat for pleasure, not for calories.

Eating—One of Life's Greatest Pleasures

This may sound contradictory, but eating for pleasure is truly a great way to savor one of life's sheer joys and still not gain weight. How can this be? The next time you go to any "all-you-can-eat" buffet, look at the really obese people and how they eat: they're shoveling the food into their mouths as if they're stoking a blast furnace, and they give no visible signs of enjoying the food they're eating. Then go into an excellent restaurant where top-quality but not necessarily large servings of delicious foods are offered. For example, go into a fine Indian restaurant and watch the people eat. We chose this example because, for many people, Indian food is the most pungent, flavorful, and delightful cuisine on earth. Now observe the person eating a dish such as *rogan josh*, an especially spicy and aromatic dish. He or she takes very small bites and savors each one by slowly chewing each bite as if it were the last on the plate. The fork is placed on the plate between bites to prolong the ecstacy of the meal. This is the essence of pleasurable eating. This person is truly eating for sensual pleasure and not for calories. The taste buds can accommodate only so many molecules at a time. The food tastes the same whether you take a small bite or stuff your mouth. The food shoveler also eats far more at his or her meal than the pleasure eater. By the time the serotonin level in the brain signals the fast eater to stop, he or she may have already consumed 4,000 calories. On the other hand, the person who eats for enjoyment savors each bite, prolongs the meal, and gives serotonin time to form in the brain and signal the eater to stop, while the food intake may be less than 1,000 calories. Bibiji Inderjit Kaur describes the eating of food in India as a metaphor for optimal living.

> Food, family, devotion, and community. The meaning of these words are intertwined in the vast cultural tapestry of India.
>
> In Indian life, among friends and in community gatherings, food is an indispensable part of socializing and an important aspect of any festivity. Food is given and accepted with an attitude of mutual appreciation. It establishes the concept of graceful give-and-take, and all other social interactions can be modeled on it.
>
> Perhaps the best way to bring the nations of the world into harmony would be to spread a dinner table that spans the globe. It would be a wonderful sight, all those different foods, cooked to perfection, with a rainbow of colors and a myriad of pleasing, tempting aromas, being shared in joy and gratitude by all the people of the world—and no reserved seating. Each one of us can start right now, in our own home, by trying foods of other lands and by sharing the recipes and experience of other peoples to forge this eternal link of body and soul—the grace of God through the gift of food.

Punishing yourself by eating only foods you dislike but think are healthy is a sure way to overeat when you are faced with your favorite dessert. The best way to control your feeling of deprivation is not to deprive yourself completely of those foods you truly enjoy. Antonia Novello, surgeon general under former president Bush, says:

> I always have said that it's possible to eat the foods you really enjoy if you eat the right amount.

The key is to eat smaller portions when you do eat these foods. If they are truly fattening, don't eat them with every meal. In fact, the key to weight control *and* pleasurable eating is "portion control."

Mary Barrett, writing in *U.S.A. Weekend*, describes the new wave of thought about eating:

> Thank goodness the obsessive '80's are over. The diet-bitten are converting to ice cream, pizza and steak. Not great globs of it, but tasteful mouthfuls. The '90's are, after all, about healthful pleasures.

This is not to negate what we have said about healthy eating. First, a healthy diet can be made very tasteful. Only a little creativity and imagination is required. Second, we do need to occasionally "indulge" ourselves. We should not be deprived of those dishes we truly enjoy, but we need to be very careful not to "overindulge."

Thus far we have concentrated on obtaining vigorous health and maximum happiness through exercise, dietary habits, and body awareness. An automobile bumper sticker seen in Indianapolis summarizes our exhortations in this chapter:

> Take care of your body—there's not a spare in the trunk.

Optimal living is characterized not by a spartan diet and a pathological program of ever-increasing exercise but by the concept of portion control in all of our life activities. As Sidney Cohen has said, "Sustained ecstasy is neurophysiologically impossible," but "prolonged pleasure" is the essence of optimal living. Taking care of and enjoying our bodies are one of life's greatest pathways to pleasure.

Orchestrating Health—You're the Conductor

Shirley Bruenjes of the Indiana University School of Nursing uses the phrase "orchestrating health" as a metaphor for taking responsibility for our own health. Each of us is the conductor, directing those aspects of our lives which contribute to the overall symphony of optimal health. We are in charge of each section of the orchestra, each one representing those activities which bring harmony and rhythm to our lives. As the conductor, we are personally responsible for the overall sound produced by the orchestra. We cannot allow ourselves to fall into the trap of blaming someone else for any discord that occurs in our lives.

Just as the 1990s is the decade of the brain, the 1980s was the decade of self-pity. Failures to experience optimal living were attributed to some variation of a dysfunctional family of origin. To achieve happiness, one need only nurture the child within and seek help through the multitude of organizations specializing in a particular dysfunctional lifestyle. Obviously, many people have received great benefits from these organizations, which in fact do emphasize self-responsibility. In the long run, we believe that the ultimate responsibility for improving our lives is placed directly on us. Once again, the great twentieth-century philosopher Calvin, in Calvin & Hobbes, has captured the mood of the resurgence of the necessity for taking direct personal control of our own lives. He and Hobbes are discussing his application for a job as an advice columnist. His first sample reflects much of the current thinking:

Stop whining and get a life, bozo.

Unfortunately, the tendency to blame anyone and everything besides ourselves for the unhappiness and unhealthiness in our lives is a universal trait, one that ultimately stands in the way of achieving our goal, whether it be happiness, success, a great body, health, or something else. The deplorable state of health care in the United States is a good example of our failure to take personal responsibility for our individual good health. This is not to imply that our health care system does not need reformation; it certainly does. But too often, we fail to take individual or personal measures to maintain our health. As we have seen, despite the unequivocal scientific evidence for the mental and physical benefits of vigorous exercise, we remain a nation of couch potatoes. Equally disturbing is the fact that with all of the equally sound research on the positive effects of sound nutrition on health, we still see cartloads of junk food going through the check-out counters at supermarkets. What about the mountains of research that show the relationship between obesity (resulting from lack of exercise and a toxic diet) and cancer, diabetes, high blood pressure, and heart disease? Yet look at the number of overweight people piling their platter with the worst kind of fattening foods at the nation's all-you-can-eat buffets. What about the thousands of people who become HIV positive every month through failure to use condoms to decrease the exchange of body fluids during sex, or through failure to use sterile syringes while injecting intravenous drugs? And most significant, what about those who continue to smoke despite their knowledge that 400,000 people die each year in the United States as a result of this habit? These deaths are accompanied by protracted illnesses, with the associated astronomical health care bills. The nation faces soaring medical costs that pose a genuine threat to the economic health of the country, at least partially due to our failure to take personal responsibility for our health and well-being. In the words of Michael Brown's song, "Don't Blame the Wreck on the Train,"

> When the gates are all down and the signals are flashing
> and the whistles are screaming in vain, and you
> stay on the tracks ignoring the facts,
> you can't blame the wreck on the train.

We do indeed have a responsibility for orchestrating our own health. We cannot wait around for "something to happen." It is up to us to *make* it happen. Too many people fall into the category of the woman in the song "Train of Life," by Blue Rose:

> I'm tired of sittin' on the side track
> Watchin' the main line run

The one phrase that best exemplifies optimal living is "Just Do It Now!" Only you can get off the side track of an unhealthy life and onto the main line of joy, happiness, and health. But you must do it now, not tomorrow. Life is what happens to you while you're planning for tomorrow. Ralph Waldo Emerson speaks eloquently about the need to enjoy optimal living now:

> Forget about It
>
> Finish every day and be done with it. You have done what you could. Some blunders and absurdities no doubt crept in; forget them as soon as you can.
>
> Tomorrow is a new day; begin it well and serenely and with too high a spirit to be encumbered with your old nonsense.
>
> This day is all that is good and fair. It is too dear, with its hopes and invitations, to waste a moment on the yesterdays.

Robert McCelland, in his book *Chance to Dance*, has a perfect description of optimal living:

Past moments are for remembering. Future moments are the source of hope. But life must be lived in the present moment. Now is the time to live, neither shackled by the past nor escaping into the future. Life does not last forever. We must learn to enjoy the moments of Grace which are given to us.

The lover and the fool live in the Now, neither enslaved by the past nor invested in the future. They live each moment, savoring its uniqueness and gracefulness. They have learned to eat and enjoy the strawberries along the way.

Rest assured, we will all get to the end of the road. When we get there, can we say, "I picked the strawberries along the way"?

Implementation

8

Celebrating Life

Our purpose is to consciously, deliberately evolve toward a wiser, more liberated and luminous state of being; to return to Eden, make friends with the snake and set up our computers among the wild apple trees.

Deep down, all of us are probably aware that some kind of mystical evolution is our true task. Yet we suppress the notion with considerable force because to admit it is to admit that most of our political gyrations, religious dogmas, social ambitions and financial ploys are not merely counterproductive, but trivial. Our mission is to jettison those pointless preoccupations and take on once again the primordial cargo of inexhaustible ecstasy. Or barring that, to turn out a good, juicy cheeseburger and a strong glass of beer.

—*Tom Robbins*, The Meaning of Life

Many have posited that our singular purpose is to fulfill human potential—to soar higher and higher until we ultimately achieve a constant ambiance of peace, love, and health. According to Abraham Maslow, former president of the American Psychological Association, human behavior is fueled by the desire for personal development. Maslow described the process of optimal growth as "self-actualization," which involves the ongoing realization of "potentials, capacities and talents, as fulfillment of mission (or call, fate, destiny or vocation), as a fuller knowledge of, and acceptance of, the person's own intrinsic nature, as an unceasing trend toward our unity, integration or synergy within the person."

The fact that humans have the capacity to even consider integrating their attitudes, values, behaviors, and sense of purpose is indeed a phenomenon worth celebrating. As we individually and collectively "consciously, deliberately" evolve toward more loving and creative beings, we observe milestones of progress. These change-stations help us to find our way, even in the most tumultuous times of planetary upheaval and personal unrest. This chapter is intended to sensitize readers to the importance of special guidance during times of transition—turning points—in our journey to wholeness. While Stage I: Mental Preparation and Stage II: Skill Development provide the basic tools for optimal living, successful utilization rests on our continuing ability to celebrate growth and development in a context of caring human relationships.

To "make friends with the snake and set up our computers among the wild apple trees," thereby promoting our evolution to a "more liberated and luminous" state, it is incumbent on us to comprehend the nature of our primal ancestry. In *The Healing Brain*, Robert Ornstein explores the link between evolution and human development. Besides walking on two legs and having a notable lack of feathers or fur, humans have a unique capacity for abstract, inventive thinking. Evolution has enabled us to grow beyond the legacy of our reptilian and mammalian past; we have developed the capability to create our own future, the most distinctive part of being human. Our special capabilities for language, perception, and consciousness are, for the most part, related to the amazing structure of the cerebral cortex. The 100 billion or so neurons—with trillions or even millions of connections—set us apart from all other species.

To grasp the concept of the amazing speed of human evolution, imagine that Earth's entire history has occurred in one solar year, with today representing December 31. Human beings would not appear until 11:45 P.M. today, and all recorded history would occur in the final minutes of that year. Given the time scale of Earth's history, humankind has developed and multiplied with unprecedented speed. In only 13 million years, humans have evolved from tree-dwelling primates, forced from their tree homes by dominant pre-chimpanzees, to a population of nearly 5 billion beings who inhabit every geography and climate on Earth, and even environments outside Earth's nurturing atmosphere. We have evolved from simple gatherers to sociable beings able to grow beyond our evolutionary inheritance to devise our own environment, celebrate our uniqueness in speech, and express our artistic spirit through abstract, inventive thinking.

How did we evolve so quickly? There is a footprint in Africa, impressed in the sand more than 3.5 million years ago, that marks the spot where human beings diverged from the rest of creation, where our ancestors first stood on two legs, not four. This seemingly simple yet monumentally important feat set into motion a whirlwind chain of events. The shift from four legs to two caused our ancestors to rely more on vision and less on smell. They could more easily see approaching danger, as well as increased opportunities for food and shelter. By shifting from time-consuming food gathering to hunting, a few hunters were able to feed several families for days. Food sharing allowed us to establish a more permanent and cooperative society.

The postural change also set in motion many physical changes. The human pelvis thickened to support additional body weight, which altered the entire process of childbirth, as the thickened pelvis decreased the size of the birth canal. Simultaneously, the human brain and head were growing larger. To adapt to these physiological changes, human beings began to be born extremely early in development. Thus, the major portion of the human brain's development occurs outside the womb, thereby endowing the external environment with a more significant role in brain development than is true for any other primate. Additionally, environmental and sociological influences in our physical and emotional world differ for each person. Thus, our individual brains are more different from each other than is the case with other primates.

All of these lightning-quick (by evolutionary standards) changes—walking, hands, pelvis, childbirth, increased brain size—occurred simultaneously, resulting in a more highly developed brain. In fact, this combination of factors has caused the human brain to evolve faster than any other organ. In only a few million years, the human brain grew from 400 to between 1,250 and 1,500 cubic centimeters, and suddenly developed the capacity for abstract thought. Our brain position also altered, by moving higher up in the skull, thus allowing the palate inside the mouth to enlarge to fill that space solely so that Cro-Magnon humans could speak better than Neanderthal ones.

With the development of language and symbols, the most sophisticated human tools, our evolutionary pace quickened with unprecedented speed. Cro-Magnons could now plan, organize, and cooperate much more efficiently. In addition to developing more sophisticated tools, shelters, and settlements, Cro-Magnons developed complex art, as evidenced by the beautiful 15,000-year-old cave paintings in Périgueux, France.

Art and language are significant milestones in human evolution because they signify a mind capable of abstraction, symbolism, and invention. Creating art is not only an abstraction of the present world but also a representation of an individual's interpretation of the universe and spiritual values. Abstract, inventive thinking has been the key to human adaptation. It ensures our survival with the creative use of tools and nurtures our spirit through art and language.

As Shakespeare wrote in *Hamlet*, "What a piece of work is a man! How nobel in reason! How infinite in faculty!" Yet Hamlet ponders suicide:

> To be, or not to be,—that is the question;
> Whether 'tis nobler in the mind to suffer
> The slings and arrows of outrageous fortune,
> Or to take arms against a sea of troubles,
> And by opposing end them?—To die,—to sleep,—
> No more; and by a sleep to say we end
> The heart-ache and the thousand natural shocks
> That flesh is heir to,—'tis a consummation
> Devoutly to be wish'd. To die,—to sleep;—
> To sleep! perchance to dream:—ay, there's the rub;
> —Act III, Scene I

While the young prince contemplates self-annihilation, Ophelia, his female counterpart, finds herself on the brink of madness. Shakespeare calls his audience to a vivid confrontation with the very meaning of life. The gut-wrenching questions that were posed in sixteenth-century Elizabethan theater echo themes that have been played across cultures since time immemorial. Indeed, life often seems "like a tale told by an idiot, full of sound and fury, signifying nothing." To glean a sense of meaning and purpose from what appears to be "a brief flicker between two eternal darknesses," humans have developed a colorful array of rituals and ceremonies, most of which focus on the significance of birth, procreation, and death. The perception of meaning begins with our senses.

Senses: The Portals of Discovery

We discover the world through our senses. Collectively, they serve as portals to tranquillity, titillation, and discovery—evolution's triggers for pleasure and fulfillment. The process is so automatic that, in the rush of our day-to-day lives, we tend to underappreciate these critical "doors of perception." Our sensory system—sight, hearing, touch, taste, and smell—is the communications network that makes us aware of the world around us. Through our senses, we break apart reality into energized bits of detail and arrange them into meaningful patterns—color, harmonies, softness, sweetness, and fragrance.

Nothing is so startling as when one of our senses goes awry. A simple cold or a callused finger is serious enough to cue our awareness to the reality of the value of our sensory system. Amazingly, when one of our senses is hampered, the others readily compensate for the limitation. Helen Keller lived a remarkable life despite her inability to see, hear, or speak. Author Diane Ackerman writes of Ms. Keller:

> One of the greatest sensualists of all time . . . was a handicapped woman with several senses gone. Blind, deaf, mute, Helen Keller's remaining senses were so finely attuned that when she put her hands on the radio to enjoy music, she could tell the difference between the cornet and the strings. . . . She wrote at length about the whelm of life's aromas, tastes, touches, feelings, which she explored with the voluptuousness of a courtesan. Despite her handicaps, she was more robustly alive than many people of her generation.

Of all our sensing abilities, sight is often considered the most vital and pleasurable way in which we observe ourselves and our world. What we regard as seeing is actually our brain's interpretation of visual images. We can close our eyes and still see splendidly colored memories. Even when we sleep, we may dream scenes in incredible detail. Because the eye is stimulated by variety, we are quickly attracted to new scenes and can easily take for granted all of the details around us.

What we see not only alerts us to our surroundings but also influences our moods and health. Research evidence indicates that gazing at tranquil scenes, such as a lake's calm water, the glow of a fireplace, or birds in a park, produces a state of relaxation. This type of low-energy activity can, at least briefly, reduce blood pressure and stress. In the hustle-bustle routine of modern living, when life's stresses seem insurmountable, one can truly find calm and tranquillity in simple visual pleasure. Getting in touch with natural beauty as nature presents itself is not only pleasing to the eye but healthy as well. Repeatedly, aquarium gazing has been shown to be beneficial in lowering hypertension and blood pressure—and in aiding apprehensive dental patients. In one study, a group of fearful dental patients gazed into an exotic aquarium for forty minutes before their procedures. They were told to relax during their operation by envisioning the peaceful image of the fish tank. The fish watchers reported a significant decrease in anxiety and discomfort during the procedure.

In the same way that sight influences our moods and health, our sense of hearing also has impressive effects on our emotional and physical well-being. The auditory messages of our surroundings reinforce our kinship with nature and with each other. We seem to have a built-in response mechanism that attracts us to certain sounds that influence our spirit and behavior.

Music is a man-made pleasure that enables us to appreciate our sense of hearing and rewards us with an aural landscape of sound. For example, music is one of the most available and powerful mood-enhancers we have. A well-orchestrated symphony has the power to induce fantasies of splendor and release brilliant figments of imagination. Music can be invigorating when we feel low, inspiring when we need motivation, and tranquilizing when we are frazzled. Whether we crave a "high" or a "low," we can adjust our mood with the intoxicating effects of music. Music also engages both our mind and our body. Heart rate, blood pressure, and stress levels can be reduced with the tranquilizing effects of soft music. Studies indicate that endorphins—the body's natural pain-relieving, pleasure-inducing chemicals—are released when we listen to upbeat melodies. The ever-popular Simon and Garfunkel song "Feelin' Groovy" describes this euphoria well: "Life, I love ya, all is groovy."

Our brain is constantly interpreting information from the environment through an intricate sensory network of nerve impulses. From birth, we never outgrow the need to be touched, hugged, and caressed. It is through our sense of touch that we first learn to respond. Numerous studies have shown that babies who are touched are more alert, active, and responsive—and grow faster and have fewer physical problems—than babies who aren't touched. Babies who receive early tactile stimulation also do well socially as they mature, and, as adults, they continue to touch. Without touching or being touched, we would all become isolated and weak.

Unlike our other senses, whose receptors are located in confined areas such as the eyes and ears, our sense of touch has its receptors located throughout the entire surface of our body. Of all our sensory organs, skin is the largest, weighing in at about ten pounds, containing receptors for pressure, vibration, temperature, and pain. In all of our senses, the receptors transmit information to our brain by way of the nervous system. As is true of vision and hearing, overexposure to our sense of touch can have a numbing effect, as it becomes insensitive to repeated stimulation.

We often touch others in the way we ourselves would like to be touched. Being touched is comforting and pleasurable, even when we touch ourselves. Think of the ways in which we touch ourselves. We play with hair strands, touch our cheek to wipe a tear, scratch our head when we're nervous, clap our hands when we're happy, or pat our stomach when it's full. We comfort and soothe ourselves by touching and extend those feelings by touching others. When we touch other people, we are rewarded with a double sensation. First, our receptors immediately interpret how a reciprocal hug feels to us; second, they then interpret how it feels to be hugging the other person. It is this mutual exchange of sensation that connects touching with our feelings.

As evidenced in studies of pets, touch can be just as therapeutic to the "toucher" as to the "touchee." One such study involved monitoring the survival rate of patients who had experienced heart attacks and whether or not pet ownership would influence their recovery. The researchers discovered that those patients who had pets that could be petted and stroked had not only a speedier recovery rate, but also a longer survival rate. The physical contact between owner and pet appears to produce mutual benefits. The pet owner receives comfort and pleasure by stroking his or her animal, and the pet, in turn, feels nurtured and accepted. Both share a sense of connection and feel less isolated.

With all the knowledge regarding the advantages of tactile stimulation, it is disheartening to admit we are raised in a society that discourages touching from the time we learn to walk. Nonetheless, we find substitutes to caress throughout our lives, such as teddy bears and domesticated animals. Our need to touch and be touched is vital and exists from birth to death. Touch is a sensual pleasure that is essential to life and to emotional well-being.

Taste and smell differ from the aforementioned senses in that they are chemical senses—they react to chemicals rather than energy. Our sense of taste can discern an array of moods, from contentment to excitement. The satisfaction we get from food can certainly affect our emotions. Every chocoholic knows the hedonistic pleasure of savoring a bite of Godiva chocolate with childlike delight.

The receptors for taste and smell work together, creating a combined effect when interpreted by the brain. When we have a cold, food seems to lose its flavor, but actually, we have only temporarily lost our sense of smell. This complementary interaction also works in reverse. The smell of vinegar from an opened jar of dill pickles may move from the nose down into the mouth, stimulating the taste buds and producing a "mouth-watering" effect. So what we refer to as smell may sometimes be taste and vice versa.

When our receptors for smell are stimulated by chemicals in the air, nerve impulses are generated to the part of the brain that involves emotions. Does the smell of freshly baked cinnamon rolls do anything for you? How about the smell of evergreens? Robert Ornstein reports that in a recent experiment, laboratory subjects were wired to physiological monitors and asked stress-provoking questions, such as "What kind of person makes you angry?" Mood, blood pressure, heart rate, respiration, and brain waves were measured. Occasionally, before the questioning, the fragrance of spiced apples was diffused into the examination room. Stress responses were modified markedly—lower blood pressure, slower breathing, greater muscle relaxation, and slower heart rate. The subjects also reported feeling happier, less anxious, and more relaxed. "In other studies the spiced apple fragrance was more effective than eucalyptus or lavender in increasing a brain wave pattern associated with a relaxed but alert state."

Once a smell has been impressed on our minds, it is rarely forgotten. The memory of the experience will fade, but reexposure to the original stimulus triggers lasting and unforgettable sensations. As one middle-aged businesswoman recalls:

I was walking through the men's department and the salesgirl handed me a sample of English Leather cologne. The second I held it to my nose, my senior prom flashed into my head and the thought of dancing all night with Tom made my heart flutter. . . . I married him years later.

Our senses are the pathways of life energy throughout our bodies. Once we become aware of the way we process our environment and identify what it is that sparks enjoyable emotions within us, we can draw on a universe of natural pleasures. Becoming aware of our senses provides the opportunity to alter our moods in positive, healthy ways.

Nerve pathways are standing by, ever ready to speed pleasure signals to our brain. From touching to teasing, from caring for others to becoming sexually aroused—the involuntary responses of the senses are on constant alert in men and women. Take our response when given a rose. Invariably, after acknowledging the initial beauty of the flower, the next spontaneous and predictable response is to bring the flower to the nose; inhale the heady fragrance in a slow, deep breath; and relax. This is often followed by touching the silky petals to more sensitive areas of the skin, such as the face, lips, or back of the hand. A rose is, indeed, a most sensual gift of nature. While its beauty is aesthetically pleasing to our sense of sight, its perfume has the power to evoke fantasies of pleasure, as the velvety touch of the petals tenderly arouse our sensual passions. Is it any wonder that we so strongly correlate roses and romance?

Fragrances inspire us. Beauty stimulates us. Touching arouses us. How rewarding it is to become aware of the experiences that spark our senses and emotions. We are exposed to a universe so abundantly filled with natural pleasures that we tend to easily overlook even the simplest forms of sensuality. "Taking time to smell the roses" may help us focus on the joys of our senses and, in return, secure our connection to each other and our world. Diane Ackerman writes:

How we delight our senses varies greatly from culture to culture. . . . [Y]et the way in which we use those senses is exactly the same. What is most amazing is not how our senses span distance or cultures, but how they span time. Our senses connect us intimately to the past . . . in ways that most of our cherished ideas never could. For example, when I read the poems of the ancient Roman poet Propertius, who wrote in great detail about the sexual response of his ladyfriend Hostia with whom he liked to make love by the banks of the Arno, I'm amazed how little dalliance has changed since 20 B.C. Love hasn't changed much, either: Propertius pledges and yearns as lovers always have. More remarkable is that her body is exactly the same as the body of a woman living in St. Louis right now. All her delicate and quaint little "places" are as attractive and responsive as a modern woman's. Hostia may have interpreted the sensations differently, but the information sent to her senses, and sent by them, was the same.

The one thing that has remained constant throughout history is human sensuality. Sensuality is the cornerstone of our being and the key to intimacy and healthy sexual relationships. Stimulation of our senses, especially touch, can convey many messages, including warmth, caring, comfort, and reassurance. Sensually, touch can be used merely for the pleasure of being close to someone. Sexually, it can open the door to arousal and lovemaking.

The sexual experience involves a blend of all our senses, but for many people, touch is the most powerful way of evoking sexual arousal. We validate each other as sensual beings by reciprocal touching. When we touch another person, we experience the warmth, smoothness, and contour of his or her body, and in return, the person being touched discovers an awareness of his or her body that serves to enhance the sexual experience. When the sexual experience involves the whole person, and both persons, pleasure and satisfaction are shared and enjoyed. The intensity of the sexual experience varies considerably from person to person, so that feelings, moods, preferences, and attitudes must be effectively conveyed as a means of strengthening the bond between partners and promoting the growth of the relationship.

Humans are unique from other animal species in that we use sex not only for procreation but also as an intimate way of bonding with another person. Intimate relationships help satisfy our need to feel connected to someone, to give and receive affection, and to develop self-esteem. Through intimacy and commitment, we develop the support systems that allow us to weather the "slings and arrows of outrageous fortune" and rise to the challenge of life's inevitable series of turning points and transitions. Intimacy and caring provide the ideal matrix for the celebration of change.

Celebrating Change: Birth, Friendship, Adulthood

Life is a journey on which we constantly face forks in the road—decisions we must make, changes we must accept. As with most of life's experiences, some turning points are anticipated and joyful, others unwelcome and problematic. Regardless of the reasons for change, the way we respond often depends on the rites and rituals we employ to commemorate these passages. If we are to find meaning in new direction, we must let go of the old and accept the new. It is not enough to physically take new steps. We must mentally and emotionally enter each new stage as well. Each passage in life must be embraced and worked through; and historically, *rites of passage* have been the method of promoting smooth transition.

Rites of passage have been studied, analyzed, and written about for centuries. Carl Jung studied these rituals from the perspective of the collective unconsciousness—"the source of faith and intuition, a wellspring of wisdom . . . to which we turn for guidance in moments of crisis."

The late Joseph Campbell took collective unconscious even further, to say that myth—the result of society's collective unconscious—"is our deep understanding of ourselves, retrieved from the dream world by our professional dreamers—prophets, shamans and priests—at our times of direst need." Campbell referred frequently to the power of the myth of the hero/heroine, which is expressed in almost all traditional initiation rites and rites of passage. It is the physical reenactment of that myth that is called ritual.

But it was the French anthropologist Arnold van Gennep who coined the phrase "rite of passage" for these rituals, describing them as "a ceremony or ritual that serves to ease the transition of individuals from one status to another, most commonly connected with birth, initiation into adulthood, marriage and death." Van Gennep went on to describe three separate stages to these rites: (1) separation (from the former status); (2) transition (a period of learning the new customs and new expectations); and (3) reintroduction (return to life in the new status, marked by a series of rituals).

Each major passage in life—birth, copulation, and death—is marked by a complicated mix of emotions, not only for the person making the journey, but for those he or she touches along the way. If any stage of these rites is not experienced, the emotional result can be devastating. In the words of anthropologist Barbara Myerhoff, "Men and women are not simply born. They are 'made' by ceremonies. Nor are they truly sexual, adult beings until certain social conditions have been fulfilled . . . and in many places, biological death is no death at all. Ceremonies must transform the corpse into a properly deceased person."

Evidence of rites of passage can be traced back through historical writings, as well as literary works of fiction. Only a few are still celebrated by certain religious and ethnic cultures in this country. In many of the so-called primitive societies, however, tribal and communal initiation rites and ceremonies are the norm and continue to maintain the vital importance they've enjoyed for centuries.

Birth

The traditional rites of passage welcoming a new baby center on two main themes: giving the child a name and formally presenting the child to his or her community or religion. In the Roman Catholic religion, one ceremony is designed to both christen (name) and baptize (welcome into the faith) the child. In this particular ceremony, the separation and transition phases are somewhat combined, as the sprinkling of the water, which washes away the child's former state of original sin, and the invocation of the Blessed Trinity are done simultaneously. This is followed by anointing the child with holy oils and lighting the baptismal candle. After the ceremony is completed, the reincorporation stage begins, as the priest raises the child and presents him or her to the congregation, naming the child and asking the church members to accept him or her into their community.

In the Jewish and Moslem faiths, circumcision is the first ritual performed at birth, while the Mormon church welcomes its youngest members with the father's blessing on the baby. The child's father is joined by his friends, who form a circle while holding the baby, each man with one hand underneath the child and the other hand resting on his neighbor's shoulder. After blessing his child ("I bless you with the peace and love of your family. I bless you with happiness in these troubled times. I bless you with the power to see the beauty in the world"), the father tells the child in his own words about the hopes and dreams he has for the newborn.

Traditional ceremonies are not exclusive to religious communities. Many Native American tribes have rituals to welcome the birth of a child, whose naming is the responsibility of the tribal elders. Canadian Blackfeet utilize a three-part ceremony in which the baby is purified (separated from the sins of the ancestors). The ritual begins with the building of a fire composed of grasses on a clay altar. The tribal elder paints the sign of the tribe on the baby's face (transition), and the ceremony ends as the elder holds the baby high toward the sun while announcing the child's name (reintroduction).

In several tribes, the women play active roles in the initiation rites of the baby. The North Yemenite mother and child are confined to the home for forty days following the child's birth, in order to avoid being accosted by devils and the evil eye. This forty-day separation and transition period is followed by a celebration of the child's reintroduction into the community.

An Australian aborigine mother prepares for her child's purification by building a fire to which she adds a stream of her breast milk, passing her baby through the smoke to eradicate the sins of their ancestors. Again, on their return to the village, a celebration takes place to welcome the baby into the community.

Friendship

Social interaction plays an important role in everyone's life. As human beings, each of us has an inborn need to feel connected to others. We thrive as separate individuals with an innate need to function as a part of a larger society that, in return, gives us our sense of safety and security. One way we fulfill our sense of human connectedness is through the friendships we develop throughout our lifetime. Whether the friendship is lifelong or short-lived, the experience strengthens our bond to humanity by filling in where family connections have been thinned by divorce, careers, and continuing social changes.

Through their understanding, tolerance, and loyalty, friends provide a buffer against stress and are a source of positive feelings about oneself. Similar values and life goals are basic for cultivating new friendships, but more important, respect for each other as unique human beings and validation of feelings are essential for the growth of the relationship. Friendships enrich our lives by causing us to feel accepted, understood, and loved. As Aristotle said, "Friendship is two bodies sharing the same spirit."

Judith Worell offers the following suggestions as "the glue that holds close friendships together":

1. Be friend-centered, not self-centered.
2. Respect each other's individuality.
3. Show compassion.
4. Share joy.
5. Offer emotional support.

Caring relationships are founded on principles of unconditional acceptance, mutual support, and respect for individual uniqueness. Real friendships allow each person to be who he or she is without any strings attached. Friends go beneath the surface, accepting things they might not understand and honoring feelings that might be left unspoken. Ideally, one's closest friend is one's lifemate.

Adulthood

Certainly there is no more traumatic period of life than adolescence, and there is no other life stage that relies so heavily on friendship. During puberty, our bodies prepare themselves for reproduction. Physiological changes occur that make intercourse, conception, and childbirth possible. Mentally and emotionally, from early adolescence throughout the rest of our lives, most of us are preparing for futures that will be shared with a partner and include giving birth to and raising the next generation of children.

Adolescence is not to be taken lightly. With hormones raging, we navigate that narrow waterway between childhood and adulthood with overwhelming confidence one second and utter fear and trepidation the next. While our peers and adult personalities tell us we should be searching for our perfect mate, our childlike psyches tell us Barbie Dolls and Ninja Turtles are still much more fun. Ambiguity is a constant companion as we seek our niche in life. How are we to decide what we want to do as adults and with whom we want to do it when we're still not ready to leave childhood behind?

The attainment of manhood is widely regarded throughout the

world as a matter of personal pride and achievement. On Truk Island, a tiny atoll in the South Pacific, men provoke each other with a popular challenge: "Are you a man? Come, I will take your life now." In East Africa, young boys from cattle-herding tribes traditionally take leave from their mothers and experience painful circumcision rites by which they become men. According to David Gilmore, author of *Manhood in the Making: Cultural Concepts of Masculinity*, "If the Samburu boy cries out while his flesh is being cut, if he so much as blinks an eye, he is shamed for life as unworthy of manhood." After completing a rich cross-cultural analysis, Gilmore concludes:

> In all these cases the tests and accomplishments involved are those that will prepare boys and youths specifically for the skills needed in adult life to support, protect and expand the living community. And it is only when these skills are mastered and displayed communally, in public, that manhood is conferred consensually upon the youth.

Yet within the period of one generation in the West, traditional routes to adulthood have become almost extinct. Confirmation, Bar Mitzvah, and Bas Mitzvah, for many, seem to belong more to the 1950s epoch of Annette Funicello and Dick Clark. Modernization has devalued such transcendent experiences, leaving ritualized expressions of alienation and distress. For many youngsters, Club Kids and teenage gangs have replaced the esprit de corps of team sports and social groups.

Many societies begin a young girl's initiation rite at the anticipation or onset of menses. In some countries, these ceremonies are conducted for several girls at the same time and often include a mock marriage with a ceremonial bridegroom.

In the Bemba tribe of Central Africa, older women have the responsibility of teaching the initiates through a series of tests designed to evaluate their feminine skills. During the process, the girls are told folktales and proverbs about the perfect wife. They learn the dangers of adultery and the risk to small children of eating food cooked by an adulteress or menstruating woman. While the girls must perform all the tasks, it is the fiancé of each girl who receives the congratulations on his future wife's performance.

The Ndembu of Northern Rhodesia emphasize male and female fertility in their initiation rites. Planning the complex ceremony begins at the first sign of puberty. The bride-to-be spends most of the first day lying under a blanket beneath a milk tree (one having white sap) while the women of the tribe dance around her. After feasting at sunset, the women carry the girl to her grass, sexually configured seclusion hut. Each carrier bears a leaf from the milk tree—a "baby"—which she races to the hut of the future grandmother.

The girl spends the next three months in isolation, visited only by her female elders, who coach her in the nuances of sex and in perfecting her erotic coming-out dance. At the end of the girl's seclusion, the teachers groom her and hide white milk-tree beads in her hair. After being ornately dressed by her women friends, the bride is feasted and hidden in the bush. She is revealed "like a spirit" and performs a variety of fertility mimes, with considerable emphasis on the providing power of women, including an act of ritual reversal—hunting—that defies the sex-role system. When the dance is over, she is carried into her husband's hut, whose upright arrow by the marriage bed exemplifies his potency. The bride keeps the white hair beads hidden until after consummation, when she shows him the prized fertility objects.

The boys' initiation ceremony is no less a fertility rite. After a night-long dance, the boys are herded to the site of the circumcision by a figure known as the Hyena, whose role is to "steal" the boys from their mothers. The boys pass through a gateway frame and tunnel of their guardians' legs, leading to the operation site and lodge area. Rebirth is symbolized by the use of a milk tree as the site of circumcision. Each boy keeps a thick stub of wood—*ankala*—to use for a pillow and chair. It represents the penis and is the cause of many laughs in the lodge.

Finally, when healed and trained in hunting and sexual competency, the novices are painted with white spots, and victoriously returned to their mothers. Their entry is sudden and confusing, so that no mother may recognize her son. After this, the circumcision lodge is burned, followed by the final initiation dance, where each ornately dressed boy performs a war dance before the chief.

Because Christian influences have been introduced in these societies, many of the details of their initiation ceremonies have been discarded over the past thirty years. For the most part, the rituals have retained several common elements, such as separation from the mother (or former stage of life), as well as a period of seclusion; introduction to the myths and "secrets" of the ancestors and instructions as to the expectations and responsibilities of adulthood; and some ceremonial reincorporation into the community. In many cases, circumcision (both male and female), scarification (the scarring of the body through a patterned series of cuts and slashes), and traditional acts of bravery are also included in these initiation rites. But regardless of the form the ritual takes, the primary intent and purpose behind the ceremonies remain the same: *to arrive at adulthood with more dignity.*

Project Self-Discovery, in Denver, Colorado, is an intensive, twelve-week transition ceremony designed to help youth who are at risk for becoming harmfully involved with alcohol or other drugs, or with other harmful lifestyles. The first week of the change process involves *Mental Preparation,* whereby youth are provided state-of-the-art information on biological, psychological, and social aspects of substance abuse and other at-risk lifestyles. The second phase, *Skill Development,* which evolves during the next eleven weeks, promotes the development of emotional, behavioral, and cultural competencies by engaging youth in artistic, recreational, and health-oriented mentorship experiences. The final *Commitment* stage requires youth to complete a wilderness journey that stresses solitude, self-disclosure, bravery, and concern for others. Family and other community members participate in a graduation ceremony that incorporates artistic and verbal statements of participants' commitment to individual, family, and social well-being.

Intimacy: Sharing the Journey

Intimacy helps to satisfy our need to feel connected to someone, to give and receive affection, and to develop self-esteem. It is these kinds of relationships that provide our support system when life gets difficult. Intimacy can best be described as a caring and trusting relationship in which thoughts, needs, and feelings can be openly expressed and unconditionally accepted. Therefore, freedom in communication is an essential aspect of an intimate relationship. Developing true intimacy requires taking risks. It means exposing our most guarded emotions and vulnerable areas to another person, who may or may not attack. But it is only through this kind of risk-taking that genuine trust and true intimacy can develop. If partners are unaccustomed to this type of emotional communication, the thought of revealing one's emotions can seem quite threatening. Many relationships must learn to allow intimacy to develop.

When emotional intimacy fails to develop or is purposely avoided, sex often becomes a goal-oriented performance. That is, sex is perceived as a single, instantly gratifying act that blocks out emotional awareness and eventually sensual awareness to the point of diminished interest in sex and/or one's partner. Sexual responsiveness declines, and any sense of intimacy is lost.

Negotiating differences in a sexual relationship requires commitment and practice. Conflict doesn't have to be viewed as a negative situation; it can instead be considered a stimulus for growth, provided both partners are working toward resolution. In *The Pleasure Bond*, Masters and Johnson explain that couples can achieve resolution of conflict by two principles they call neutrality and mutuality. Neutrality means that each partner respects the good intentions of the other and trusts that those intentions are genuine and sincere. Each partner takes personal responsibility for his or her actions and sexual responses. If a couple is "to have a good physical relationship, each must strive to be responsive to the other, not responsible for the other."

The principle of mutuality defines the sexual interaction between two persons, whether by speech or actions, in the "spirit" of working toward a mutual cause. The common goal of partners in a healthy sexual relationship is to discover and accept what pleases each other, to be sensitive to individual needs and differences, and to be committed to working together toward mutual satisfaction, knowing that their sexual preferences will not always match perfectly.

The key here is a commitment to full communication of our honest feelings in order to remain attuned to our partner's needs as well as our own. We have a responsibility to accept the special uniqueness of each other as individuals and to honor each other's wants or desires in a way that enables us to satisfy our sexual needs. This is the mutually cooperative effort that will sustain a healthy and successful sexual relationship.

Some fundamentally important aspects are involved in developing and maintaining a healthy sexual relationship. First, honesty and a commitment to full communication form the cornerstone to building trust and intimacy. When problems arise, it is important to find resolution rather than solution. That is, both partners must be committed to openly expressing their needs and feelings in a caring way and to accepting those ideas with concern and respect for individual likes and differences. Freedom of expression and effective communication are essential elements of an intimate relationship and are the key to conflict resolution. We are not automatic interpreters of body language or semiaudible verbal cues. It takes effort and assertiveness for couples to discover what is best for each other. Expressing thoughts and feelings as clearly as possible is the responsibility of both partners. If clear communication is lacking, neither partner will be able to respond effectively and satisfaction will slip into frustration.

Second, partners must never bring "old garbage" into a new relationship. If, for instance, one person has been betrayed in a previous relationship, it is crucial to future relationships to work on feelings of hurt and trust so that this sort of unfinished business is not brought into the new relationship. Expecting that a previous negative experience is going to repeat itself is destructive to the current relationship. When a partner brings "old garbage" into a relationship, it invalidates the other partner's uniqueness as an individual. It puts a new person in an old scenario, which is dangerous. One might as well put a death sentence on the new relationship. Sometimes it is difficult to get in touch with old feelings and previous experiences to honestly look at ourselves, but if old feelings aren't somehow resolved, we get stuck. It's the things we choose not to think about that keep us from becoming healthy and growing as individuals. Honesty with ourselves is basic to being honest in a relationship.

Third, it is important to the success of the relationship that both persons remain individuals with their own interests. Maintaining independence within a relationship gives us the capacity to set goals, pursue new interests, and function well as an individual as well as a partner. The self-actualization and personal satisfaction that are enjoyed enhance the quality of the relationship and make each partner more interesting to the other. Pursuing outside interests not only encourages self-awareness, but also promotes personal autonomy, which prevents partners from becoming overly dependent on each other. When autonomy fails to develop before a serious relationship is formed, dependencies are simply transferred from parents to partners.

Last, sexual commitment involves sexual responsibility. That is, each of us takes responsibility for clearly expressing our sexual wants and needs, and for remaining attuned to our partner's wants and needs. The responsibility, however, does not end with the mutual satisfaction of the sexual encounter; rather, it includes the obligation of full commitment of both partners to the responsibility of pregnancy and birth control. Every potential outcome of sexual interaction is the mutual responsibility of both partners. According to Masters and Johnson:

> Total commitment, in which all sense of obligation is linked to mutual feelings of loving concern, sustains a couple sexually over the years. In the beginning, it frees them to explore the hidden dimensions of their sexual natures. . . . Then, when carrying the inescapable burdens that come with a family and maturity, they can turn to each other for the physical comforting and emotional sustenance they need. . . . Finally, in their later years, it is the enduring satisfactions of their sexual and emotional bond that committed husbands and wives find reason enough to be glad that they still have another day together.

The development of commitment, intimacy, and responsibility serves as the framework for maintaining healthy, caring relationships and is the foundation for future roles throughout the rest of our lives. The roles we experience throughout our lifetime are continually shifting. Being single, being part of a couple, being part of a committed relationship—all require a shift in emotional intensity as we make the transition from one role to another. Most people agree that sustaining a satisfying relationship with another person takes a great deal of emotional investment and energy, which may be difficult for many people, but we continue to search for closeness and intimacy even though there may be no clear-cut path to follow.

For the majority of Western society, marriage becomes the context in which intimate, committed relationships develop. In the United States today, more than 90 percent of men and women will marry in their lifetime. As we become secure in the knowledge that another person will share our journey, is boredom the inevitable result? According to David Schnarch, author of *Constructing the Sexual Crucible*, the answer is quite to the contrary:

> Marriage is a crucible. Marriage creates gut-wrenching, sinew-testing situations that force people to grow up in a way that makes possible, very, very intense sex and eroticism.

Through working with older couples, Schnarch found that there is a group—which he refers to as "the blessed few"—who can successfully integrate sexuality and spirituality. These persons report a sensation of time stopping when they are having sex and often talk about feeling that some spiritual force has sent them their partners. These couple report what Schnarch calls "wall-socket" sex:

> Wall-socket sex is jolting. If you want to have an idea of it, have sex with your eyes open. Never look away from your partner, and look him right in the eye. Or really slow down your touch—enough so that you can actually *feel* your partner. People develop the ability to touch without feeling. Just think about how you hug your mother or uncle for a demonstration of touching without feeling. The trouble is, for a lot of us, that also applies to our spouse.

But one must be adequately prepared for the "sexual crucible." If not, society will remain heir to only a "blessed few" who can combine sexuality and spirituality.

In *Women Who Run with the Wolves*, Clarissa Pinkola Estes discusses how women are often ill-prepared to face the challenge of intimacy:

> One of the central and most potentially destructive issues women face is that they begin various psychological initiation processes without initiators who have completed the process themselves. They have no seasoned persons who know how to proceed. When initiators are incompletely initiated themselves, they omit important aspects of the process without realizing it, and sometimes visit great abuse on the initiate, for they are working with a fragmentary idea of initiation, one that is often tainted in one way or another.

Carol Rovito-Heckman, mother of two teenage children, had the difficult experience of journeying toward intimacy with neither adequate preparation nor social support. She views the transition as a haphazard—and therefore harrowing—rite of passage, from which she emerged as a person capable of independent functioning, only now ready to participate in a genuinely intimate relationship. Had she been privy to a meaningful ritual for the transition, much of her suffering might have been avoided.

My own divorce took place four years ago, after an emotionally destructive, fourteen year marriage. None of the knowledge I accumulated as a child could have prepared me for that marriage, because nothing in my childhood prepared me to be an effective adult. As an adolescent, I cautiously teetered on that very fine line between adolescence and adulthood until, at the age of seventeen, I met my future husband—someone to define my role and be an adult for me when I couldn't handle it.

For fourteen years, I lived a very childlike adult existence, never having to make a decision for myself. I was told [by my husband] what to think, what to feel, what to like, and what to dislike. I was told what to wear, what to eat, when and how long to sleep. I was instructed on where to go and where not to go, to whom I should talk and what to say when I did talk to them. I accepted this as a child accepts because I had no base of self-esteem and no formal awareness of when I had become an adult and was capable of making my own decisions.

After my husband left, I continued to allow him to make my decisions. He told me what I needed to do with the rest of my life, what my limitations were, what kind of man I should look for, and when I should start looking. He controlled my spending, my relationship with my children, and even my social life. He assured me that if I just listened to him and did what he told me to do, *he* would make sure I was OK.

Finally, after six long months of this seclusion into what I thought was reality, after hearing all of the myths and the legends he chose for me to believe, I experienced my own private initiation and passage into adulthood. My husband insisted he had paid me enough since the separation began and would pay no more money until he was ordered by the court to do so. I had no skills, no education, no career goals, so was unable to support myself or my kids. I headed to the bank to draw from what little savings I had, but discovered I also had no funds—he had frozen them. As I left that bank, some voice inside of me screamed, "You can no longer be a child—you are an adult. Act like one!" I knew without a doubt that now *I* would have to make sure I was OK. If my kids were to have a future, it would be up to me to see that they had one. No one could or would make my decisions— I would make them myself.

It took me a very long time to experience my passage into adulthood, and the road since hasn't always been an easy one. I have, at times, mourned the simplicity of my former life and its lack of personal responsibility. I have, at times, been almost overwhelmed with the fear of being alone. And then reality returns as it did one morning in early December, almost two years ago.

On a day when my kids were home from school and we all decided to sleep in, I woke up at about 9:00 in a state of panic. For a few minutes, I was back in that marriage and terrified that my husband would find out I had slept so late and wasn't getting anything done. My mind went over and over what I would say to him by way of explanation, until it finally occurred to me I was no longer married to him—I was no longer under his abusive control. It was entirely up to me how long I slept, what I accomplished on a daily basis, if, in fact, I chose to accomplish anything. The relief was almost overwhelming. My life was now my own, and I was almost hysterically happy about that. I was an adult, I could make my own rules, and I was going to truly love the freedom of making my own decisions.

I can't say that each day since then has been full of that some joyful hysteria. It has sometimes been a very steep, uphill battle. But those few moments of fear and the relief that followed were perhaps the most effective rite I could have experienced to mark the emotional transition into my new life as an adult.

Sharing Knowledge, Wisdom, and Experience

As humans approach midlife, an emotional shift occurs: a previous view of life diminishes, as the true concept of our mortality sinks in. Robert Michels, chairman of the Psychiatry Department at Cornell Medical School, describes this shifting view of one's life as a refocusing of personal hopes and dreams to more "symbolic extensions of the self," such as one's family, one's community, or a cause.

Erik Erikson explained this "generativity" transition as occurring when the level of happiness in our life is determined by the concept that we begin to share the knowledge, wisdom, and experiences of our life with younger generations, who now look to us as their mentors and role models. This is the time of life when compassion and deepening personal relationships become more intense, and our emotional lives become enriched as a result of this caring, sharing integration.

Caring, belonging, and feeling connected to other human beings are needs that begin at birth and are lifelong. The continuity of transgenerational involvement is an important aspect of human connectedness, through which older generations influence younger generations, as well as the reverse. For many older adults, younger generations are a source of pride, comfort, and concern, persons with whom they can share their past and present lives. As role models and mentors, older generations can significantly influence young people as they determine their goals and ambitions. In general, older generations offer a source of wisdom, reflection, and guidance to younger generations who have not yet chosen their life's course.

As children, we learn values, attitudes, and behaviors from family, friends, and all other social contacts. Whether or not a child develops a caring, compassionate attitude depends largely on the quality of nurturing and the values and attitudes of the role models to which the child is exposed. When cooperation, helpfulness, compassion, and generosity are modeled and valued, and children are respected and loved as unique individuals, caring relationships develop and continue throughout life.

In the early nineteenth century, French philosopher Auguste Comte identified a behavior that exemplified an unselfish concern for the welfare of others and coined the term *altruism*. Today we refer to *altruism* as an active sense of concern for helping and caring for others without expecting anything in return. Altruists do not limit their unselfish deeds to family and friends, rather, they extend their natural and spontaneous concern to the rest of society. This compassionate and generous nature is the foundation of caring relationships.

The renowned twentieth-century psychologist Abraham Maslow viewed altruistic behavior as a brilliant reflection of personal psychological well-being. The kindness and compassion of the altruistic person are grounded in the understanding that all human life is interconnected and that helping each other is fundamental to maintaining our bond with humankind. Maslow also believed we are born with an affinity for altruism, compassion, love, and friendship that develop with the care and nurturing we receive as children.

The support and understanding present in a caring relationship produce a pervasive sense of well-being and simultaneously reward us with a sense of having received nourishment from nurturing others. Helping others nourishes our self-esteem by promoting a feeling of genuine appreciation from others and makes us feel we have made a difference. Because of the rapidity of changes in our society, breakdown of the American family and fragmentation of the community have left us with an inner hunger to feel connected to and a part of a larger social body. Doing something to make a difference gives new meaning to life by instilling within us a sense of fulfillment and satisfaction that may have been lacking. Caring about and helping others reward us with a positive attitude, which in turn gives us the advantage of better mental as well as physical health.

In a recent series of interviews with volunteers in various community organizations, an overwhelming majority indicated that the time and energy they invested in voluntarism gave them more personal satisfaction then they ever expected. They reported that their involvement in volunteer work gave them a double reward—the satisfaction of benefiting those in need and the experience of the "helper's high"—exhilarating and euphoric sensations felt as a direct result of helping others. It's been said that nobody can help another without helping him- or herself, which may stand as the ultimate foundation for the Golden Rule. Giving time and consideration to a serious social matter outside home or work expands the volunteer's world in positive ways.

"Helper's high" is described in a recent editorial by Dean Edell:

> Years ago I volunteered to help teach at a Head Start school for disadvantaged kids. On my first day there I noticed a small Hispanic girl with large eyes standing by herself in the corner. Her teachers told me they worried about her because she wouldn't play with the other kids. I decided to make getting to know her my special project. With the help of time and persistence we managed to become good friends, even though her English was poor and my Spanish worse. She started smiling back at me and reached for my hand whenever we strolled around the school grounds. I still remember how good I felt after my visits with her. It's clear to me that helping another human being can produce a high that's almost indescribable. Several studies have found that people who regularly help others feel better afterward. . . . The idea that helping is good for your health seems like a win-win situation to me. I often think of that little girl and wonder if she could

possibly have gotten anywhere near the benefits that I enjoyed from our relationship.

Helping others and caring about those in need are powerful lessons that begin early. The possessive and aggressive nature that defines the character of a two-year-old is also accompanied by prosocial behavior and compassion. When very young children are observed, the need to respond to distress in others becomes quite apparent. When an infant cries for its mother, it's not unusual for a two-year-old sibling to comfort the baby until help arrives. By reinforcing this behavior with their own compassionate actions, parents teach children to become more caring and altruistic. It is the nature of the young child to do good things for others, and it is the wise parent who encourages this natural desire for kindness and compassion so the child will grow into a caring adult.

In addition to a sense of pride and accomplishment, the world of voluntarism offers opportunities to learn new skills while sharing knowledge and expanding social experiences, thereby creating new bonds with others and maintaining a sense of human connectedness. In addition, the volunteers broaden their personal perspectives of understanding life from other angles. As the generation of "baby boomers" reaches middle age, an encouraging view of priorities is emerging, emphasizing compassion, enrichment of emotional ties, and development of deeper, personal relationships.

History is filled with caring, compassionate individuals who make it their life ambition to dedicate their efforts to the service of humanity. In New York City, Clara Hale is known simply as Mother Hale to hundreds of drug-addicted and AIDS babies whom she cares for each year, giving away her $19,500 salary. Her humanitarian efforts have inspired hundreds of other communities around the country to set up similar programs for unwanted infants so desperately in need of care. On a more global basis, the compassionate work and charity of Mother Theresa are recognized worldwide. In 1979, she was awarded the Nobel Peace Prize for her devoted efforts to relieve the sufferings of the poor, sick, and dying in the slums of Calcutta. A true humanitarian, she is venerated by people of all beliefs. Her dedication to the service of the homeless poor led her to establish the Missionaries of Charity, whose present community includes 700 members working on five continents.

From the turn of the century until 1965, the dedication to serving humanity was perhaps most brilliantly exemplified by philosopher, physician, musician, clergyman, missionary, and theology writer Albert Schweitzer. As a young man, Schweitzer based his philosophy on the significance of "reverence for life"—a worldview that all creatures are one—which evoked a deep sense of obligation to serve humanity. He became a medical missionary, established a leper colony, and built a large hospital in Gabon, where he treated thousands of Africans. Martin Luther King, Jr., writes:

> . . . the most durable power in the world . . . love is an absolute necessity of the survival of our civilization.

The Ultimate Celebration

Death is perhaps the most fear-inducing word in the English language. With few exceptions, there is little about it that we control—neither the time, place, nor method of dying. And we know nothing about what takes place after it occurs. Contradictory stories abound, involving idyllic utopias and fiery pits of eternal damnation. Those who have survived near-death experiences speak of hearing voices and following warmth and bright lights. Some embrace the concept of reincarnation, intellectualizing about the famous people they knew or even were in their former lives, and wistfully anticipate who they will be when they are reborn. The bottom line is that we don't know what happens—death is still a mystery.

The ceremonies that accompany this final passage, especially in our culture, are designed both to facilitate the deceased's spiritual passing into the afterlife and to ease the survivors' emotional acceptance of that passing. We pay homage to our dead in personalized ceremonies that depict the mourners' beliefs as well as the beliefs and wishes of the deceased. Further, in many ways, these ceremonies emphasize not only the way the deceased lived but the manner in which he or she died.

For example, the tone at the recent funeral for a ninety-six-year-old man was decidedly peaceful and serene. The ritual was clearly designed to be a celebration of the life of this much-beloved man, and each member of his large extended family took part. His love and concern for the homeless and hungry were commemorated by food gifts placed by each of his great-grandchildren in baskets surrounding the church's altar. His love for his family was remembered in stories and poems recited by each of his children and grandchildren. And finally, his love and devotion for his wife were represented by the pall that covered his casket: an heirloom quilt, given to him and his wife when they moved to Colorado sixty years earlier. As his grandson explained during the service, the quilt was first used to celebrate this gentleman's journey to Colorado and was now used to celebrate his journey to his Father in heaven.

In sharp contrast was the funeral service for a twenty-seven-year-old man who, following a childhood and adolescence marked by his parents' divorce, family dysfunction, rebellion, drug abuse, and alcoholism, took his own life after a failed robbery attempt. This young man's funeral bore no resemblance to the older gentleman's. There were few expressions of love or cherished memories. The primary focus of the eulogy was to ask people to pray for his soul and forgive him if he had caused them any pain during his brief life. The final passage of this man's life was anything but a celebration of that life—it was almost an apology for it.

Certainly most of the rites of passage involving death fall somewhere between these extremes, as do the rituals and customs of other societies. Primitive cultures seem to focus more on their belief in spirits, both good and evil ones. The Dineh (Navajo) believe the deceased's spirit becomes a temporary, evil ghost. The dead person's shoes are reversed to confuse the *chindi* (ghost) so it cannot find its way back to his or her body. The name of the dead is not uttered, for fear the *chindi* will hear its name and answer the unintentional invitation.

In Bucharest, a young woman who dies before she has married is buried in a bridal gown, with a small doll placed beside her in the coffin to represent her unborn children. In addition, her family chooses a bridesmaid to be present at the funeral—all in an effort to protect her against the possibility of becoming an "unfilled soul."

Another theme is the continuation of life, with death being a doorway to the next state. In Africa, where death is considered a simple status change, the deceased remains very much present in the community, where he or she will continue to be a source of guidance and wisdom. To that end, the person's body is buried with life's essentials—food, clothing, cooking and eating utensils—all for the comfort and use of his or her body as it passes into the "other world."

In Yunan Province, China, some mourners prostrate themselves as the funeral procession passes, while others set off noisemakers and firecrackers in a effort to ward off evil spirits. And in the same vein, African Bushmen bury their dead with heavy stones piled both on top of the corpse and again on top of the grave in an effort to prevent ghosts from coming back to haunt them.

Whatever the method or manner of burial, in traditional societies and cultures, the passing of a loved one is marked and celebrated. We are humans—we need the pomp and circumstance. Even in death we celebrate ourselves.

Birth, childhood, adolescence, intimacy, marriage, divorce, retirement; turning forty, fifty, or sixty; grieving the loss of a relationship or the death of a loved one, or anticipating one's own death—each of these events is an emotional passage that must be fully experienced in order to leave behind one's former stage and peacefully embrace the new. Developing a ritual that celebrates these and other passages, and makes the transition a healthy and fulfilling one, should be of utmost importance to all of us. If we work as communities to reintegrate ceremonies of change into our culture, we may be able to make a difference in the lives of many of our adolescents and young adults—and subsequently, all our lives. It is the entire community that raises a child.

Epilogue

My late grandmother, it seemed, had somewhat of an obsession about time and its passing. One of my strongest memories of this remarkable woman is hearing her steady stream of time-oriented clichés when she felt we weren't making the most of each moment—"Time is money," "Time is of the essence," "Time marches on," "A stitch in time saves nine"—Grandma used them all and seemed to have one at her disposal no matter which time-wasting crime we had committed. In fact, as children my cousins, sisters and I would place bets on which pearl of wisdom would fall from her lips on any given occasion, with the winner being excused from the after-dinner chores.

I was never sure at the time where Grandma got these little phrases—did she actually hear them somewhere or did she devote hours to making them up? But as I have gotten older, I have been reminded again and again of Grandma's quotes and have learned that the only thing we can be sure of is that time goes by very quickly and, like the tide, "waits for no man."

What Grandma failed to warn us about were the changes that would take place in our lives during the speedy passage of time, and the emotions that would both enrich our lives and, at times, break our hearts with each of those changes. Such passages are both natural and plentiful, but it's the time and attention we give to those passages that determines the ease with which we sail through them.

—Carol Rovito-Heckman
unpublished diary

References and Notes

Introduction
Say Yes to Natural Highs

Carson, Rachel. "The Sense of Wonder" *Omni*. Greensboro, NC, January 1989, p. 33. (Article by Jane Bosveld.)

Dumas, Alan. See Parker, Cindy.

Maugham, W. Somerset (1944). *The Razor's Edge*. Doubleday, Doran & Co.: Garden City, NY.

Siegal, Ronald (1989). *Intoxication: Life in Pursuit of Artificial Paradise*, E. P. Dutton: New York.

Watterson, Bill. "Calvin & Hobbes" Kansas City: Universal Press Syndicate, 6/10/90, 2/2/92, 2/5/92.

Milkman, H. and Sunderwirth, S. "The Chemistry of Craving" *Psychology Today,* October, 1983.

Parker, Cindy (Sept. 1992). From a personal interview with Alan Dumas, feature writer, Rocky Mountain News, Denver, CO.

World Health Organization (1964). Basic Documents (15th Edition), p. 1, Geneva, Switzerland.

Chapter 1
Blueprint for Fulfillment

Borysenko, Joan (1987). *Minding the Body, Mending the Mind*. Addison Wesley: Reading, MA.

Cohen, Sidney (1988). *The Chemical Brain: The Neurochemistry of Addictive Disorders,* Irvine, CA: Care Institutes.

Eliot, T.S. (1970). "Hysteria" *Collected Poems 1909–1962,* 11th Printing. New York: Harcourt, Brace & World, Inc.

Emerson, Ralph Waldo (1921). Essays and Poems of Emerson. New York: Harcourt Brace.

Fernstrom, J.D., Faller, D.V., Shabshelowitz, H. (1975). Acute reduction of brain serotonin and 5-HIAA following food consumption: correlation with the ratio of serum tryptophan to the sum of competing amino acids. *J. Neural. Transm.* 36(2):113–21.

Gardner, Howard (1983). *Frames of Mind: The Theory of Multiple Intelligences,* New York: Basic Books.

Hughes, J. (May 2, 1975). Isolation of an endogenous compound from the brain with pharmacological properties similar to morphine. *Brain Res.* 88(2):295–308.

Kazantzakis, N. (1960). *The Last Temptation of Christ.* Simon & Schuster: New York.

Kosterlitz, H.W. and Hughes, J. (July 1, 1975). Some thoughts on the significance of enkephalin, the endogenous liquid. *Life Sci.* 17(1):91–6.

Lincoln, Abraham (1842) in Szasz, Thomas (1974). *Ceremonial Chemistry.* Doubleday & Co., Inc.: New York.

Maddi, Salvatore and Kobasa, Suzanne (1984). *The Hardy Executive: Health Under Stress.* Homewood, IL: Dow Jones-Irwin.

Marc, D. (1984). "Understanding Television" *The Atlantic Monthly.* Institute of Mental Health, (1982), pp. 33–44.

Ornstein, R. and Sobel, D.S. (1989). *Healthy Pleasures.* Addison Wesley.

Pilecki, Tom (12/4/88). "Art in the South Bronx" *Sixty Minutes.*

Rosellini, Lynn (1992). "Breeding Olympic Stars" *U.S. News & World Report.* February 17, 1992, pp. 48–57.

Werner, Emmy (1989). "Children of the Garden Island" *Scientific American.* April.

Wurtman, R.J. and Fernstrom, J.D. (1974). Control of brain serotonin by the diet. *Adv. Neurol.,* 5:19–29.

Chapter Two
Nurturing the Healthy Child

Attinger, Joelle (February 29, 1988). "When the Sky's the Limit." *Time Magazine.*

Berk, Laura E. (1991). *Child Development,* 2nd Edition. Boston: Allyn and Bacon.

Berkman, Joanna J. (Spring, 1983). "For Spacious Skies" *The Amicus Journal.*

Brazelton, T. Berry and Cramer, Bertrand G. (1990). *The Earliest Relationship: Parent, Infants and the Drama of Early Attachment.* Reading, MA: Addison-Wesley.

Bredekamp, Sue and Rosegrant, Teresa (Eds.) (1992). "Reaching Potentials: Appropriate Curriculum and Assessment for Young Children." Washington, DC: National Association for the Education of Young Children.

Burroughs, William S. (1953). *Junkie.* New York: Ace Books.

Conger, John J. (1991). *Adolescence and Youth,* 4th Edition. New York: Harper Collins.

Dennis, W. (1973). *Children of the Creche.* New York: Appleton-Century-Crofts.

Eron, L.D. (1982). "Parent-child interaction; televised violence and aggression of children." *American Psychologist* 37(2):197–211.

Fulghum, Robert (1988). *All I Really Need to Know I Learned in Kindergarten: Uncommon Thoughts on Common Things.* New York: Villard Books, Div. of Random House.

Fraiberg, Selma (1959). *The Magic Years: Understanding & Healing the Problems of Early Childhood.* New York: Scribner.

Gibran, Kahlil (1973). "On children." *The Prophet.* New York: Alfred A. Knopf.

Glantz, L.H. (July/August 1991) "Criminal prosecution of pregnant drug users." *Addiction and Recovery.*

Goldstein, Herman (1977). *Policing a Free Society.* Massachusetts: Balinger Publishing Company.

Groening, Matt (1990). "The Simpsons" Fox Television Network.

Johnson, Earvin "Magic" (3/25/92). "A Conversation with Magic: A Nickelodeon Special."

Kagan, Jerome (1988). "The Mind: Part II—Development." Alexandria, VA: PBS Video.

Kiell, N. (1967). *The Universal Experience of Adolescence.* Boston: Beacon Press.

Mudd, John (1984). *Neighborhood Services: Making Big Cities Work.* New Haven, Yale: University Press.

Restak, Richard (1988). "The Mind: Part II—Development." Alexandria, VA: PBS Video.

Satir, Virginia (1972). *People Making.* Palo Alto, CA: Science and Behavior Books.

Schull, William J. (1988). "The Mind: Part II—Development." Alexandria, VA: PBS Video.

Shinkle, Florence (1990). "Circus Flora" *St. Louis Post-Dispatch.*

Singer, J.L. (1975). *The Inner World of Daydreaming.* New York: Harper and Row.

Stokols, Daniel (1992). Establishing and Maintaining Healthy Environments: Toward a Social Ecology of Health Promotion. *American Psychologist,* 47(1):6–22.

Unknown Author (1992). "Don't Wait Until You See Me," *Chicago Tribune.*

Weidlein, Marianne (1991). *The Day We Speak Peace Handbook.* Boulder, CO: Aimari Press.

White, Burton L. and Myerholb, Michael D. (1992). "What is Best for the Baby" *The Infants We Care For.* Washington, DC: NALYC (National Association for the Love of Young Children).

Wilson, James Q. and Kelling, George L. (February, 1989). "Making neighborhoods safe." *The Atlantic.* Boston, MA.

Chapter 3
The Chemical Brain: Molecules and Mood

Blake, William (1982). In *The Complete Poetry and Prose* of William Blake, Edited by David Erdman. Garden City, NY: Anchor Books.

Blum, K. (1991). *Alcohol and the Addictive Brain: New Hope for Alcoholics from Biogenetic Research.* New York: Macmillan.

Cloninger, C.R. (1987). "A Systematic Method for Clinical Description and Classification of Personality Variants." *Archives of General Psychiatry,* V 44(6):573–588.

Cohen, S. (1988). *The Chemical Brain.* Irvine, CA: Care Institute.

Crick, Francis H.C. (1992). "Profile: Francis H.C. Crick, The Mephistopheles of Neurobiology," *Scientific American.* February, 1992.

Delgado, P.L., Charney, D.S., Price, L.H., Aghajanian, G.K., Landis, H., and Haninger, G.R. (1990). "Serotonin Function and the Mechanism of Antidepressant Action." *Archives of General Psychiatry* V 47(5):411–418.

Diaz, Bernal. In Idell, Albert, Ed. (1956). *Bernal Diaz Chronicle: The True Story of the Conquest of Mexico.* Garden City, NY: Doubleday.

Durden-Smith, J. and deSimone, D. (1983). *Sex and the Brain.* New York: Arbor House.

Goldstein, A. (1982). Oral Presentation at the Sixth Annual Summer Institute on Drug Dependence, Colorado Springs, Colo.

Howela, Lisa. "Jeffrey Dahmer." Indianapolis Star, 2/1/92.

Hughes, J., et al. (1975). "Identification of Two Related Pentapeptides From the Brain with Potent Opiate Agonist Activity." *Nature* 258:577–579.

Kalus, O., Asnis, G. and Van Praag, H. (1989). "The Role of Serotonin in Depression." *Psychiatric Annals* 19(7):348–353.

McGinn, C. (1991). *The Problem of Consciousness.* Oxford, UK; Cambridge, MA: B. Blackwell.

Meltzer, H. (1990). "Role of Serotonin in Depression." *Annals of the New York Academy of Sciences,* V 600, 486–500 (October).

Ornstein, R. and Sobel, D. (1989). *Healthy Pleasures.* New York: Addison-Wesley.

Olds, J. and Milner, P. (1954). "Positive reinforcement produced by electrical stimulation of septal area and other regions of the rat brain." *J. Comp. Physiol. Psychol.,* 47:419.

Routtenberg, Aryan (1978). "The Reward System of the Brain." *Scientific American* 239(5):154–164.

Steiger, Rod. In Thomas, Bob, "Steiger's Back and Willing to Act," Indianapolis Star, 2/6/92.

Styron, W. (1990). *Darkness Visible—A Memoir of Madness.* New York: Random House.

Sunderwirth, S. and Milkman, H. (1991). "Behavioral and Neurochemical Commonalities in Addiction." *Contemporary Family Therapy* 13:421–433.

Thomas, Lewis L. (1974). "Fear of Pheromones," *Lives of a Cell: Notes of a Biology Watcher.* New York: Viking.

Van Gogh, Vincent. In Hulsker, Jan, Ed. (1971). *Van Gogh "Diary"—The Artist's Life in His Own Words and Art.* New York: William Morrow.

Waterson, Bill. "Calvin & Hobbes." Kansas City: Universal Press Syndicate, 2/2/92.

Wurtman, R.J., and Wurtman, J.J. (1989). "Carbohydrates and Depression." *Scientific American,* January, 68–75.

Chapter 4
Using Your Inner Resources

Alpert, Richard (1978). "Coming Down" *Be Here Now*. New York: Hanumen Foundation, Crown Publishing: New York, NY.

Csikzentmihalyi, Mihaly (1990). *Flow: The Psychology of Optimal Experience.* Harper & Row: New York.

Davidson, R.J. and Schwartz, G.E. (1976). "The Psychology of Relaxation and Related Staztes: A Multi-process Theory" *Behavior Control and Modification of Physiological Processes*. New York: Prentice-Hall.

Gardner, H. (1992), cited in Goleman, D. et al., *The Creative Spirit*. New York: Dutton.

Goldstein, Joseph (1976). *The Experience of Insight: A Natural Unfolding—A Simple and Direct Guide to Buddhist Meditation*. Utility Press: CA.

Goleman, Daniel (1988). *The Meditative Mind: The Varieties of Meditative Experience*. Los Angeles: Tarcher, St. Martin's Press.

Holmes, Richard and Rahe, Richard. "Scale of Stresses" cited by Suzanne Oullette Kobasa in *American Health Magazine,* September, 1984.

Huxley, Aldous (1960). "Ordinary Experiences—What a Piece of Work is Man." The Pacific Radio Archives.

Huxley, Aldous (1970). *The Doors of Perception*. New York: Harper & Row.

Kobasa, Suzanne Ouellette (1984). "How Much Stress Can You Survive?" *American Health Magazine*. New York: Reader's Digest Corp., September.

Lilly, John (1972). *Center of the Cyclone*. Julian Press: NY.

Montague, Margaret P. (1917). *Twenty Minutes of Reality: An Experience with Some Illuminating Letters Concerning It by Margaret Prescott Montague*. New York: Dutton.

Moore, Thomas (1992). *Care of the Soul*. HarperCollins: New York.

Rainey, Frank. "Multiple Intelligence Profile Indicator." In press.

Selye, H. (1969). "Stress: It's a G.A.S." *Psychology Today* 2(4):pp. 25–26, 56.

Snyder, Soloman H. (1986). "Drugs and the Brain," *Scientific American Library*. New York: W.H. Freeman and Co.

Walker, Alice (1983). *The Color Purple*. New York: Harcourt Brace Jovanovitch.

Whitman, Walt (1958). "Leaves of Grass." New American Library: NY.

Woodman, Marion (1982). *Addiction to Perfection*. Inner City Books: Toronto.

Note: "Hardiness Inventory," "Scales of Stresses," and "Pathways to Hardiness" were originally published in *American Health Magazine*, September, 1984, pp. 64–77, "How Much Stress Can You Survive?" by Suzanne Oullette Kobasa.

Chapter 5
Finding the Balance

Ball-Rokeach, S.J., Rokeach, M. and Grube, J.W. (1984). *The great American value test: influencing behavior and belief through television. Psychology Today*, November.

Bauch, Aubrey (1980). Personal communication.

Bandura, A. (1982). Self-efficacy mechanisms in human agency. *American Psychologist,* 37, pp. 122–147.

Bandura, A. Self-efficacy mechanism in physiological activation and health-promoting behavior. In J. Madden, S. Matthysse & J. Barchas (Eds.) *Adaptation, Learning and Affect.* New York: Raven, in press.

Bennett, H.L. et al. (1986). Preoperative instruction for decreased bleeding during spine surgery. *Anesthesiology, 65(3A),* A245. [30w]

Benson, Herbert (1989). *Your Maximum Mind.* Avon Books: New York.

Castaneda, Carlos (1968). *The Teachings of Don Juan: A Yaqui Way of Knowledge.* Berkeley and Los Angeles: University of California Press.

Cousins, Norman (1979). *Anatomy of an Illness as Perceived by the Patient: Reflections on Healing and Regeneration.* New York: Norton, pp. 68–69.

Cushman, Ann (1992). "Are You Creative?" *Utne Reader.* Minneapolis, MN, March–April.

Estes, Clarissa P. (1989). *Journeys into Creativity: Myth and Stories About the Creative Fire.* Sounds True Recordings, Boulder, CO.

Gardner, H. (September, 1982). "Giftedness: Speculations from a Biological Perspective" *New Directions for Child Development: Developmental Approaches to Giftedness and Creativity, No. 17,* D. Feldman, Ed. San Francisco: Josey-Bass.

Goleman, Daniel (1988). "Erikson in his own old age, expands his view of life." *New York Times,* "Science Times" 6/14/88, pp. 13, 16.

Goleman, D., Kaufman, P., and Ray, M. (1992). *The Creative Spirit.* New York: Dutton.

Griffin, Jean Latz (1992). "Humor helps teen girls accept pregnancy." *Denver Post,* Denver, CO, 4/2/92.

Harner, Michael (1990). *The Way of the Shaman,* Tenth Anniversary Edition. San Francisco: Harper San Francisco.

Jung, Carl (1964). *Man and His Symbols.* Doubleday: New York.

Kadloubovsky, E. and Palmer, G.E.H. (1969). *Early Fathers from the Philokalia.* London: Faber & Faber.

Kadloubovsky, E. and Palmer, G.E.H. (1971). *Writings from the Philokalia on Prayer of the Heart.* London: Faber & Faber.

Kaiser, Robert Blait. "The Way of the Journal," *Psychology Today.* March 1981.

Kraft, Kenneth (Ed.) (1988). *Zen, Tradition and Transition, 1st Edition.* New York: Grove Press.

Lorig, K., Laurin, J. & Holman, H. (1984). Arthritis self-management: A study of the effectiveness of patient education for the elderly. *The Gerontologist* 24.

Lowie, Robert H. (1952). *Primitive Religion.* New York: Grosset and Dunlap.

Maslow, A.H. (1971). *The Farther Reaches of Human Nature.* New York: Penguin Books.

Ornstein, R. and Sobel, D.S. (1987). *The Healing Brain.* New York: Simon and Schuster.

Ornstein, R. and Sobel, D.S. (1989). *Healthy Pleasures.* Reading, MA: Addison Wesley.

Peterson, C. and Seligman, M.E. (June, 1987). "Explanatory Style in Illness." *Journal Personality and Social Psychology* 55(2).

Peterson, C., Seligman, M. and Vaillant, G.E. (1988). "Pessimistic Explanatory Style is a Risk Factor for Physical Illness: a 35-year longitudinal study." *Journal Personality and Social Psychology*.

Progoff, Ira (1980). *The Practice of Process Meditation*. New York: Dialogue House.

Progoff, Ira (1975). *At a Journal Workshop*. New York: Dialogue House Library. (Dialogue House Associates, 80 E. 11th St., Suite 305, New York, NY 10003–6008 is the administrative headquarters for the Intensive Journal Program)

Rokeach, M., Ball-Rokeach, S.J. (1989). "Stability and change in American value priorities, 1968–1981." *American Psychologist, Vol. 44, No. 5*. May, 1989.

Santas, Gerasimos Xenophon (1979). *Socrates, Philosophy in Plato's Early Dialogues*. London and Boston: Routledge & K. Paul.

Sinclair-Gieben, A.H.C. & Chalmers, D. (1959). Evaluation of treatment of warts by hypnosis. *Lancet, ii*, pp. 480–482.

Singer, D.G. and Singer J.L. (1990). *The House of Make Believe: Children's Play and the Developing Imagination*. Cambridge, MA: Harvard University Press.

Sobel, D.S. (1990). The placebo effect: Using the body's own healing mechanisms. In R. Ornstein & C. Swencionis (Eds.), *The Healing Brain: A Scientific Reader*. New York: Guilford.

Sobel, D.S. (1990). The Optimism Antidote: When Belief Becomes Biology. Presentation at *The Healing Brain: Using the New Science of Mood Medicine*. San Francisco, November 17, 1990.

Spanos, N.P., Stenstrom, R.J. & Johnston, J.C. (1988). Hypnosis, placebo, and suggestion in the treatment of warts. *Psychosomatic Medicine* 50:245–260.

Wallis, C. (1983). "Stress: Can We Cope?" *Time*. New York, June 6, 1983, pp. 48–54.

Wanberg, K.W. and Milkman, H.B. (1992). "The Personal Pleasure Inventory. Denver, CO: The Center for Interdisciplinary Studies, Inc.

Whitman, Walt (1992). *The Creative Spirit*, "There was a child went forth every day," as quoted by Goleman, D., Kaufman, P. and Ray, M. New York: Dutton.

Williams, R.B. (1987). Psychological facts in coronary artery disease: Epidemiologic evidence. *Circulation*, 72 (Suppl):I117y–I123.

Williams, R.B. (1989). *The Trusting Heart: Great News About Type A Behavior*. New York: Time Books.

Chapter 6
Orchestrating Fitness

Beale, N. and Nethercott, S. (1986). "Job-loss and Health—the influence of age and previous morbidity." *Journal of the Royal College of General Practitioners* 36:261–264.

Blake, M.J., Stein, E.A., and Vomachka, A. (1984). "Effects of exercise on brain opioid peptides and serum LM in female rats." *Peptides* 5:953–958.

Brothers, J. (1989). "Do you have enough fun?" *Parade Magazine,* July/August, 37–39.

Brown, J.D. and Lawton, M. (1986). "Stress and well-being in adolescence: The moderating role of physical exercise." *Journal of Human Stress* 12:125–131.

Brown, Jr., Jackson (1991). *Life's Little Instruction Book.* Nashville, Tennessee: Rutledge Hill Press.

Caspersen, C.J., Powell, K.E., and Christenson, G.M. (1985). "Physical activity, exercise and physical fitness." *Public Health Report* 100:126–130.

Cooper, Edward (1992). "Physical inactivity as a risk factor." *Newsweek,* November 21.

Dishman, R.K. (1988). *Exercise Adherence.* Champaign, Illinois: Human Kinetics Books.

Dunn, A.L., and Dishman, R.K. (1991). "Exercise and the Neurobiology of Depression." In *Exercise and Sport Sciences Reviews,* edited by John O. Holloszy, p. 41–97. Philadelphia: Williams & Wilkins.

Folkins, C.H. (1976). "Effects of physical training on mood." *Journal of Clinical Psychology* 32:385–388.

Gottlieb, B. ed. (1992). *Training the Body to Cure Itself.* Emmaus, PA: Rodale Press.

Greist, J.H. (1984). "Exercise in the treatment of depression." *Coping with mental stress: The potential and limits of exercise intervention.* Washington, DC: National Institute of Mental Health.

Greist, J.H. et al. (1978). "Running Through Your Mind." *Journal of Psychosomatic Research* 22:259.

Gutfeld, G. (1992). "Flex Rx." *Prevention,* February.

Harmatz, M.G. (1985). "You are as fat as you think." *Shape,* April.

Harris, S.S., Caspersen, C.J., DeFriese, G.H., and Estes, H. (1989). "Physical activity counseling for healthy adults as a primary preventive intervention in the clinical setting: Report for the US Preventive Services Task Force." *Journal of the American Medical Association* 261:3590–3598.

Hutchinson, M.G. (1985). *Transforming Body Image: Learning to Love the Body You Have.* Trumansburg, NY: Crossing Press.

Long, B.C. (1984). "Aerobic conditioning and stress inoculation: A comparison of stress-management interventions." *Cognitive Therapy and Research* 8:517–542.

Long, B.C. (1985). "Stress-management interventions: A 15-month follow-up of aerobic conditioning and stress inoculation training." *Cognitive Therapy and Research* 9:471–478.

McCann, I.L. and Holmes, D.S. (1984). "Influence of aerobic exercise on depression." *Journal of Personality and Social Psychology* 46:1142–1147.

Meyers, D.G. (1992). The Secrets of Happiness." *Psychology Today,* July/August.

Morgan, W.P. (1985). "Affective beneficence of vigorous physical activity." *Medicine and Science in Sports and Exercise* 17:94–100.

Morgan, W.P. (1987). *Exercise and Mental Health.* New York: Hemisphere Publishing Corporation.

Paffenbarger, R.S., Wing, A.L., and Hyde, R.T. (1978). "Physical Activity as an Index of Heart Attack Risk in College Alumni." *American Journal of Epidemiology* 108:166.

Roth, D.L. and Holmes, D.S. (1985). "Influence of physical fitness in deterring the impact of stressful events on physical and psychological health." *Psychosomatic Medicine* 47:164–173.

Sachar, E.J., Asnis, G., Halbriech, Nathan, R.S. and Halpern, F. (1980). "Recent studies in the neuroendocrinology of major depressive disorders." *Psychiatric Clinics of North America* 3:3113–3126.

Sinyor, D., Golden, M., Steinert, Y. and Seraganian, P. (1986). "Experimental manipulation of aerobic fitness and the response to psychosocial stress: Heart rate and self-report measures. *Psychosomatic Medicine* 48:324–337.

Slattery, M.L. et al. (1990). "Physical activity, diet, and risk of colon cancer in Utah." *American Journal of Epidemiology* 128:989–999.

Swanbrow, D. (1989). "The Paradox of Happiness." *Psychology Today,* July/August.

Thoren, P. et al. (1990). "Endorphins and exercise: physiological mechanisms and clinical implications." *Medicine and Science in Sports and Exercise* 22:417–428 (August).

Chapter 7
Eating as a Healthy Habit

Barrett, M.E. (1990). Go ahead—Indulge." *USA Weekend,* November 9.

Blue Rose (Unknown Author). "Train of Life." Tree Publishing Co., Inc.: Nashville, TN.

Brown, Michael. "Don't Blame the Wreck on the Train" *Songs of Recovery II.*

Brown, Michael. "I Want It All" *Songs of Recovery II.*

Bruenjes, S. "Orchestrating Health." In press.

Cohen, S. (1988). *The Chemical Brain.* Irvine, CA: Care Institute.

Jesse, Kathy Wyde. (1990). "Food for thought." *Indianapolis Star,* September 20.

Kline, N. (1974). *From Sad to Glad.* New York: Ballantine Books.

McCelland, R. (1986). *Chance to Dance: Risking a Spiritually Mature Life.* St. Louis, MO: Chalice Press.

Novello, A. (1990). "You can eat healthy." *Parade Magazine,* November 11.

Toufexis, Anastasia (1992). "The New Scoop on Vitamins," *Time,* April 6, 1992.

Unknown Author (1992). *Consumer Reports.* October, 1992.

Wurtman, J. (1982). "Nutrients that modify brain function." *Scientific American* 245(4):50–59.

Chapter 8
Celebrating Life

Ackerman, Diane (1990). *A Natural History of the Senses.* New York: Random House.

Alsford, D.B. (1985). "Pacific Northwest Indians" *Man, Myth and Magic, Illus-*

trated Encyclopedia of Mythology, Religion and the Unknown, Vol. 9. New York: Marshall Cavendish.

Berger, K. (1990). *The Developing Person Through the Life Span.* New York: Worth.

Byer, C., Shainberg, L. and Jones, K. (1985). *Dimensions of Human Sexuality.* Dubuque, IA: Wm. C. Brown.

Campbell, Joseph with Moyers, Bill (1988). *The Power of Myth.* Doubleday: New York.

Comte, Auguste (1936). *Cours de Philosophie Positive.* Larousse: Paris.

Crooks, L. (1989). "Volunteer Workers: Our Greatest Asset" *Modern Maturity.* Lakewood, CA: American Association of Retired Persons, Apr/May, 1989.

Davis, John. "Wilderness Rites of Passage" *Gnosis,* No. 11, Spring, 1989.

Davis, J. and Pevny, R. (1989). "Sacrifice and Purification Ceremony for a Rite of Passage" *Gnosis,* No. 11, Spring, 1989.

Douglas, Mary (1985). "Menstruation" *Man, Myth and Magic,* Vol. 7. New York: Marshall Cavendish.

Edell, Dean (1991). "The Helper's High" *The Edell Health Letter.* Sausalito: Hippocrates Partners, April.

Eisenberg, N. (1992). *The Caring Child.* Cambridge, MA: Harvard University Press.

Elkin, A.P. (1985). "Australia: Myth and Magic of the Aborigines" *Man, Myth and Magic,* Vol. 1. New York: Marshall Cavendish.

Estes, Clarissa P. (1992). *Women Who Run With the Wolves: Myths and Stories of the Wild Woman Archetype.* New York: Ballantine Books.

Ewen, D. (1992). "Albert Schweitzer" *World Book Encyclopedia.* ILL: World Book, Inc.

Forge, Anthony (1985). "New Guinea: Keeping the Balance of Creation" *Man, Myth and Magic,* Vol. 7. New York: Marshall Cavendish.

Gilmore, David (1991). Manhood in the Making: Cultural Concepts of Masculinity. Yale University Press. New Haven, Conn.

Gluckman, Max (1985). "Rites of Passage" *Man, Myth and Magic,* Vol. 9. New York: Marshall Cavendish.

Goleman, D. (1990). "Compassion and Comfort in Middle Age" *New York Times.* New York: New York Times Syndication Corp., February 6, 1990, pp. C1–C14.

Greer, Germaine (1992). *The Change: Women, Aging and the Menopause.* New York: Alfred A. Knopf.

Hunt, M. (1990). *The Compassionate Beast.* New York: Wm. Morrow and Co., Inc.

Huxley, Francis (1985). "Brazil" *Man, Myth and Magic,* Vol. 2. New York: Marshall Cavendish.

Jackson, J.A. (1985). "Initiation" *Man, Myth and Magic,* Vol. 5. New York: Marshall Cavendish.

King, Martin L., Jr. (1992). "Love, Struggle, and Excellence: Quotations from Martin Luther King, Jr." *Ebony.* Chicago, IL, January.

Knaster, M. (1991). "The Good that Comes from Doing Good" *East West*. Nov.–Dec.

Kopecky, G. (1991). "Are You a Good Friend? *Redbook*. New York, September 1991.

Lynch, L. (1992). "Who's News" USA Weekend, *Denver Post,* May 29–31, 1992, p. 2.

Martin, Herbert L., Jr. (Fall 1988). "Running Wolf: Vision Quest and the Inner Life of the Middle School Student" *Holistic Education Review*.

Martin, Herbert L., Jr. (1978). *Conduct Disorders of Childhood and Adolescence: A Behavioral Approach to Assessment and Treatment*. New York: Wiley.

Maslow, Abraham H. (1964). *Religions, Values and Peak Experiences*. New York: Penguin Books.

Maslow, Abraham H. (1968). *Toward a Psychology of Being, 2nd Edition*. New York: Van Nostrand Reinhold Company.

Masters, W.H. and Johnson, V.F. (1970). *The Pleasure Bond*. Boston: Little, Brown.

Michels, Robert, and MacKinnon, Roza A. (1971). "The Psychiatric Interview in Clinical Practice," *Saunders*. Philadelphia.

Myerhoff, Barbara and Simic, Andei (1978). *Life's Career and Aging: Cultural Variations in Growing Old*. Beverly Hills, CA: Sage.

Newman, B. and Newman, P. (1991). *Development Through Life: a Psychosocial Approach*. Pacific Grove, CA: Brooks/Cole.

Ornstein, R. and Sobel, D. (1989). *Healthy Pleasures*. Reading, MA: Addison-Wesley.

Project Self-Discovery is a four-year demonstration project, funded by the Center for Substance Abuse Prevention, Harvey Milkman, Ph.D., Project Director, 899 Logan Street, Suite 207, Denver, CO 80203.

Radke-Yarrow, M., Scott, P. and Zahn-Waxler, C. (1973). "Learning Concern for Others" *Developmental Psychol*. 8, 2:240–260.

Richmond, Douglas R. (1989). "The Legal Implications of Fraternity Hazing" *NASPA Journal,* Vol 26, No. 4. Summer, 1989.

Robbins, Tom (1991). *The Meaning of Life: Reflections in Words and Picture on Why We Are Here,* David Friend and the Editors of Life. Boston: Little Brown.

Santrock, J. (1986). *Life-Span Development*. Dubuque, IA: Wm. C. Brown.

Schnarch, David M. (October, 1992). "Moving away from sex as aerobics . . . " *Mirabella*.

Schnarch, David M. (1991). *Constructing the Sexual Crucible: An Integration of Sexual and Marital Therapy*. New York: W.W. Norton.

Stoddard, A. (1989). "Cherishing Our Friends" *McCall's*. New York: March, 1989.

Turner, Edith (1992). "Tapping the World's Ritual Resources for Our Troubled Youth: Ways to Give Adulthood to Adolescents in New York State" *Rites of Passage Symposium*. Albany, State Assembly.

Turner, Edith and Blodgett, William (1988). "The Carnivalization of Initiation in

Zambia" *The Official Journal of the Association for the Study of Play*, Vol. 1, No. 3.

Van Biema, David (1991). "The Journey of Our Lives" *Life*. New York: October 1991.

Van Gennep, Arnold (1960). *Rites of Passage*. University of Chicago Press.

Weissbourd, B. (1991). "How Children Learn to Care" *Parents Magazine*. New York: August 1991.

Wellard, James (1985). "Bushmen" *Man, Myth and Magic*, Vol 2. New York: Marshall Cavendish.

Wellard, James (1985). "Africa: You are useless, you gods!" *Man, Myth and Magic*, Vol. 1. New York: Marshall Cavendish.

Worrel, Judith (1989). *Adolescent as Decision-Maker*. San Diego: Academic Press.

Young, Frank W. (1987). "Rites of Passage" *Encyclopedia Americana*, Vol. 23.

Acknowledgments

The authors would like to thank Lyn Wickelgren, Chairperson of the Department of Psychology at Metropolitan State College of Denver, and Paul Bippen, Director of Indiana University–Purdue University at Indianapolis, Columbus campus, for their insightful comments, encouragement, and professional support. Alan Prendergast is much appreciated for his skill at bringing this work to a higher level of writing clarity. We would also like to thank Laura Mershon for her research endeavors; Lynne Sullivan for her editorial comments; and Fran Billington, Jeanette Barker, and Michelle Redifer for their editorial assistance and manuscript preparation. Carol Rovito Heckman and Donna Masoni made invaluable conceptual and literary contributions to Chapter 8. Finally, we would like to thank Paula J. Nicholas for her skill and patience in rendering the illustrations in Chapter 3.

Index